MCQs for the PLAB Examin

MCQs for the PLAB Examination

Kavita Dutta MBBS

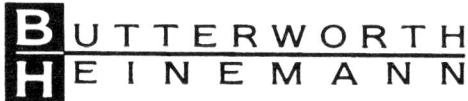

OXFORD BOSTON JOHANNESBURG MELBOURNE NEW DELHI SINGAPORE

Butterworth-Heinemann
Linacre House, Jordan Hill, Oxford OX2 8DP
225 Wildwood Avenue, Woburn, MA 01801-2041
A division of Reed Educational and Professional Publishing Ltd

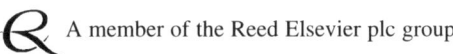 A member of the Reed Elsevier plc group

First published 1998

British Library Cataloguing in Publication Data

A catalogue record for this book is available from the British Library

ISBN 0 7506 4004 9

Typeset by E & M Graphics, Midsomer Norton, Bath
Printed and bound in Great Britain by Biddles Ltd, Guildford and King's Lynn

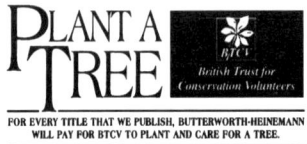

Contents

Acknowledgements

Mr Paul Gartell MS FRCS, Consultant Surgeon, Royal Hampshire County Hospital, Winchester, UK

Dr Stefano Olivieri FRCPsych., Consultant Psychiatrist, Royal Hampshire County Hospital, Winchester, UK

Preface

When I arrived in the UK, I realized how little I knew about the PLAB test although I had decided to sit the test some time back. I had to spend some time familiarizing myself with the test and the modes to prepare for it. I realized that there were only a few books on the market to help prepare for the examination and wished there were more. With a low pass rate in the test I always felt candidates could benefit immensely from practice papers, especially consisting of material from past examinations. I was fortunate to be able to compile a collection of MCQs from past PLAB tests which many of my helpful friends had collected and prepared on MCQs topics frequently repeated in the test. These MCQs are presented in 15 papers in this book. I must stress that all the MCQs in this book cover oft-repeated themes in the PLAB test and should help candidates pass the MCQ paper.

The idea behind this book and the motivation to do it came from my husband who has been a constant encouragement during the preparation and I am thankful to him. I must not forget my friend Dharminder Saroha who has supported me throughout my PLAB ordeal. My gratitude also extends to Mr Gartell, Dr Olivieri and Dr Meeran for helping realize this book.

Lastly, my thanks go to Ms Hannah Tudge and the team from Butterworth-Heinemann who made this book possible.

Kavita Dutta

Introduction

MCQ technique

How to get the most out of this book

All the MCQs in this book are based on actual questions that have appeared in the past PLAB tests. There is the possibility that some of the questions are repeated in part in different sections.

As in most MCQ examinations, certain areas or topics are commonly examined. Going through the topics that are covered by the MCQs in this book would be extremely helpful for the examination. In particular, consulting the topics in standard textbooks would be useful and thinking of ways in which MCQs could be framed out of these topics.

Timing

In the PLAB examination 60 MCQs have to be attempted in 90 minutes In all there are 300 stems (each MCQ having five). This means that one would have about one and a half minutes per question. In reality, there will be much less time per question because a revision may be required to make sure you have marked all questions in the right boxes and to attempt left-over questions.

To guess or not

For every MCQ correctly answered you score 1 point and for every incorrectly answered question you score minus 1. Hence answering many questions incorrectly can bring down one's score tremendously. This seems fine as long as you know the answer to the question with a high degree of confidence. When you are not sure or only vaguely familiar with the question the decision arises – to guess or to leave the question unanswered.

Some examinees are good guessers and some are terrible at it. It may be prudent to find out where your limits of guessing lie. One way of doing this is to attempt a mock paper. Mark your answers in three columns (ie. either high confidence, medium confidence or low confidence). When you have checked your score, calculate the percentage of answers of medium and low confidence that you scored. This will give you an idea of how good at guessing you are; whether you lose or gain marks by doing so.

Attempting the paper

Everyone has their own individual style of answering the MCQ paper which they feel confident about. A common technique used by many examinees is described below.

At the first go attempt all the MCQs you are confident of answering. Having done so quickly calculate how many stems of MCQs you have attempted. If you have attempted more than 200 stems at this point, you have probably done well and there may not be a need to do too many of the rest. Now go through the paper again and attempt the questions where you can make an educated guess or have to spend some time thinking about the answer. Wild guesses are probably best avoided.

The pass mark in an MCQ exam varies greatly and depends on the relative performance of the candidates. So, hope that you are doing better than the candidate next to you! It is hence difficult to predict how many questions need to be answered to be reasonably confident of passing although, some say 200 out of 300 stems is a safe minimum.

Common MCQ terminology

One *must* be familiar with terms used in MCQs otherwise, in spite of knowing the answers, there is a possibility of getting them wrong. The following are common terms used in MCQs and their generally accepted meanings.

Characteristic: means that it is of diagnostic significance; its absence might make one doubt the diagnosis.

Typical: means a feature you would expect to be present. It is similar to a characteristic feature.

Recognized: a 'recognized' feature is one that has been reported, but may be not be characteristic of that condition.

May: 'may' questions are usually true.

Majority, most, usually, common: are usually similar in meaning and would indicate above 50%.

Invariably: means 98–99% of the time.

Rarely, usually, uncommonly, infrequently: usually means less than 5% of the time.

Specific feature: means pathognomic for that condition and does not occur elsewhere.

Is common: is usually a poorly coined term and means more than 50%.

Is associated with: means more common than a chance association.

Always, never: are usually false. These are poor terms and hence rarely encountered in MCQs.

Avoiding common errors

There are some common avoidable errors one has to be aware of;

- Make sure you mark your MCQ in the right column in the answer sheet.
- Make sure all the 'don't know' boxes are marked where appropriate.
- Read the stem very carefully and understand the question.
- If you do not know a particular MCQ which sounds difficult, do not panic; leave it out and come back to it later. If you have already answered many questions, you may not need to do it at all. Tough questions are often meant for the toppers (unless you are one!).
- Do not just assume that examiners are trying to trick you. Avoid torturing yourself searching for hidden meanings, as this is more likely to hinder your decision making.
- Maintain momentum through the paper; time can be important.

Structure of the PLAB test

Overseas qualified doctors are normally required to pass a test of proficiency in English and of professional knowledge and skill before they can begin their first appointment in the United Kingdom for which limited registration is required. For this purpose the PLAB test is held. The test is conducted by the Professional and Linguistic Assessments Board (PLAB) on behalf of the General Medical Council, UK. The pattern of the PLAB test has recently been subject to change.

The existing pattern
There are two components of the examination, as outlined below.

1. Use of English component. To pass this the candidates have to achieve the required score stipulated by the GMC in the International English Language Testing System examination (IELTS). This examination is held at various centres across the world. For information about the IELTS test please contact the nearest British Council Office in your country.
2. Medical component. This comprises:
   • a multiple choice question examination;
   • a clinical problem-solving examination;
   • a photographic material examination;
   • part of an oral examination.

The new pattern
From early 1998, the PLAB test will be divided into two parts. Part 1 will be composed of the three written papers of the existing medical component of the test (i.e. the MCQ examination, the clinical problem-solving examination and the photographic material examination). Part 2 of the test will take the form of an objective clinical structured examination.

Only those candidates who have passed part 1 will be eligible to take part 2. Sessions of PLAB part 1 will be held in the UK and some overseas centres starting with India. In India these sessions are to be held in Mumbai (Bombay), Calcutta, Chennai (Madras) and New Delhi. The first session of part 2 is due to be held in the UK in April 1998.

All candidates who have not successfully completed the PLAB test by the end of March 1998 will have to take part in the new part 1 and part 2 system. All those candidates who have previously passed the medical component of the test from September 1995 onwards will be exempt from part 1 of the PLAB test for a period ending on the 1 January 2000. Thereafter they will be required to pass both part 1 and part 2 of the test.

Further information regarding the PLAB test can be obtained from: PLAB Test Section, General Medical Council, 178 Great Portland Street, London W1N 6JE, UK. (Tel. 0171 915 3548/3549; Fax. 0171 915 3565).

References

The following are some standard and useful references for the PLAB test. The list is by no means exhaustive but indicates books which are commonly read by junior doctors in the UK and are deemed useful.

1. Chamberlein, G. (1993) *Obstetrics by Ten Teachers.* Edward Arnold, London.
2. Chamberlein, G. (1995) *Gynaecology by Ten Teachers.* Edward Arnold, London.
3. Collier, J. A. B., Longmore, J. M. and Hodgetts, T. J. (1995) *Oxford Handbook of Clinical Specialties.* Oxford University Press, Oxford.
4. Hope, R. A., Longmore, J. M., Hodgetts T. J. and Ramrakha, P. S. (1994) *Oxford Handbook of Clinical Medicine.* Oxford University Press, Oxford.
5. Kumar, P. and Clark, M. (1994) *Clinical Medicine.* W. B. Saunders, London.
6. Mann, C. V. (1995) *Bailey and Love's Short Practice of Surgery.* Chapman and Hall, London.

Paper 1 Questions

1. Characteristic features of endometriosis include:
a) Dysmenorrhea.
b) Dyspareunia.
c) Subfertility.
d) Amenorrhea.
e) Menorrhagia.

2. Rheumatoid arthritis may be associated with:
a) Pleural effusion.
b) Pericarditis.
c) Subcutaneous nodules.
d) Carpal tunnel syndrome.
e) Myocarditis.

3. Features of posterior dislocation of the hip include:
a) Sciatic nerve injury.
b) Flexion, abduction and external rotation of the leg.
c) Avascular necrosis of the head.
d) Requires open reduction.
e) Weight bearing after 3 weeks.

4. The following are true of congenital dislocation of the hip at birth:
a) Asymmetrical creases in the thigh are found.
b) Is diagnosed by Barllow's/Ortolane's test.
c) Is diagnosed by ultrasonography.
d) Trendenlenburgh test is positive.
e) Decrease in abduction and extension of the hip is found.

5. Features of supracondylar fracture include:
   a) Common in children.
   b) Median nerve palsy can occur.
   c) Damage to brachial artery can occur.
   d) Reduction in full flexion of hand.
   e) Malunion can occur.

6. The following can undergo malignant change:
   a) Achalasia cardia.
   b) Ulcerative colitis.
   c) Melanosis coli.
   d) Familial polyposis.
   e) Crohn's disease.

7. In bone remodelling:
   a) Parathyroid hormone causes bone resorption.
   b) Increased alkaline phosphatase is an index of osteoclastic activity.
   c) Increased calcium is an index of osteoblastic activity.
   d) Osteoblasts produce osteoid.
   e) Osteoclasts cause bone resorption.

8. In the accelerated phase of the first stage of labour:
   a) Epidural anaesthesia can cause delay in labour.
   b) Cervical dilatation of more than 1 cm per hour occur.
   c) Syntocinon is not indicated.
   d) The head should be engaged.
   e) Membranes may be ruptured.

9. Congenital conditions of the bowel are:
   a) Achalasia cardia.
   b) Meckel's diverticulum.
   c) Melanosis coli.
   d) Hirchsprung's disease.
   e) Polyposis coli.

10. Increased serum amylase can be found in:
   a) Perforated duodenal ulcer.
   b) Diabetic ketoacidosis.
   c) Uraemia.
   d) Acute pancreatitis.
   e) Cystic fibrosis.

11. Olfactory hallucination may be seen in:
   a) Schizophrenia.
   b) Petit mal epilepsy.
   c) Temporal lobe epilepsy.
   d) Amenorrhoea.
   e) Allergic rhinitis.

12. The following can cause epileptic fits:
   a) Water intoxication.
   b) Adenoma sebaceum.
   c) Hypoparathyroidism.
   d) Hypocalcaemia.
   e) Hyponatraemia.

13. Characteristic features of the syndrome of inappropriate ADH secretion are:
   a) Polyuria.
   b) Hyponatraemia.
   c) Hypernatraemia.
   d) Fits.
   e) Elevated urea.

14. The following are true of persistent glycosuria in pregnancy:
   a) Serum glucose of more than 8 mmol is diagnostic of diabetes mellitus.
   b) Glucose of less than 6 mmol excludes diabetes mellitus.
   c) Serum glucose of more than 10 mmol is an indication for GTT.
   d) Increased GFR is a cause.
   e) Reduced tubular reabsorption of glucose is a feature.

15. Features of prolactin secreting microadenoma include:
a) Increase in size during pregnancy.
b) Impotence.
c) Galactorrhoea.
d) Amenorrhoea.
e) Bromocriptine is indicated for treatment.

16. Cerebrospinal fluid protein of more than 1.5 g/l is indicative of:
a) Multiple sclerosis.
b) Guillain–Barre syndrome.
c) Acoustic neuroma.
d) Viral meningitis.
e) Spinal tumour.

17. Charcot joints may be found in:
a) Poliomyelitis.
b) Leprosy.
c) Syringomyelia.
d) Diabetes mellitus.
e) Syphilis.

18. The following are recognized features of hypoparathyroidism:
a) Tetanus.
b) Tetany.
c) Abdominal pain.
d) Fits.
e) Renal stone.

19. Osteomalacia is a recognized feature of the following:
a) Coeliac disease.
b) Post-gastrectomy.
c) Vitamin D deficiency.
d) Regional ileitis.
e) Ulcerative colitis.

20. Features of Crohn's disease may include:
a) Erythema nodosum.
b) Pyoderma gangrenosum.
c) Fistula and fissures.
d) Granuloma.
e) Carcinoma of the colon.

21. Drugs of proven value in supraventricular tachycardia are:
a) Amiodarone.
b) Captopril.
c) Disopyramide.
d) Verapramil.
e) Lignocaine.

22. Fine needle aspiration cytology is useful in the diagnosis of the following:
a) Carcinoma of the tongue.
b) Thyroid carcinoma.
c) Breast carcinoma.
d) Testicular tumour.
e) Submandibular gland.

23. The following are true of medullary carcinoma of thyroid:
a) May produce calcitonin.
b) It is a hormone dependent tumour.
c) It arises from parafollicular cells.
d) May be sporadic or associated with MEN syndrome.
e) Mostly treated with partial thyroidectomy.

24. Sore tongue can be found in deficiency of:
a) Folic acid.
b) Vitamin B.
c) Niacin.
d) Iron.
e) Ascorbic acid.

25. Pharyngeal pouch:
   a) Can present as a visible swelling in the posterior triangle of the neck.
   b) Is situated between the inferior and middle constrictors.
   c) Can cause aspiration pneumonitis.
   d) Is a cause of dysphagia.
   e) Can be treated by endoscopic surgery.

26. Pulsus alternans:
   a) May be found in left ventricular failure.
   b) Is readily diagnosed by ECG.
   c) Can be a feature of constrictive pericarditis.
   d) Can be detected with a sphygmomanometer.
   e) Is associated with change in pulse volume.

27. Features of diabetic autonomic neuropathy include:
   a) Gangrene of the foot.
   b) Impotence.
   c) Postural hypotension.
   d) Diarrhoea.
   e) Sweating of feet.

28. Recognized complications of diabetes mellitus are:
   a) Sixth cranial nerve palsy.
   b) Vitreous haemorrhage.
   c) Renal calculi.
   d) Retinopathy.
   e) Nephropathy.

29. Features of renal cell carcinoma include:
   a) Lump in the loin.
   b) Polycythaemia.
   c) Varicocele.
   d) Pyrexia of unknown origin.
   e) Haematuria.

30. Polycystic disease of the kidney:
   a) Is an autosomal dominant condition.
   b) Positive family history can be found.
   c) Can present with haematuria.
   d) May cause hypertension.
   e) Predisposes to renal cell carcinoma.

31. Human chorionic gonadotrophin:
   a) Is produced by the corpus luteum.
   b) Is a steroid.
   c) Has the same biological activity as luteinizing hormone.
   d) Is an exclusive product of the placenta.
   e) The alpha-subunit is characteristic of human chorionic gonadotrophin hormone.

32. Anencephaly is associated with:
   a) Face presentation.
   b) Prolonged pregnancy.
   c) Premature labour.
   d) Shoulder dystocia.
   e) Multiple pregnancy.

33. Pathological reduction of placental blood flow may be found in:
   a) Uterine hypertonus.
   b) Pre-eclampsia.
   c) Aorto-caval compression.
   d) Epidural anaesthesia.
   e) Abruptio placenta.

34. Endometrial carcinoma is associated with:
   a) Ovarian dysgerminoma.
   b) Intermenstrual bleeding.
   c) Obesity.
   d) Hypertension.
   e) Polycystic ovarian disease.

35. In disseminated intravascular coagulopathy:
   a) Fibrinogen level is reduced.
   b) Fibrin degradation products are increased.
   c) Factor eight is increased.
   d) Platelets are reduced.
   e) Morphological abnormality of red blood cells is found.

36. Features of liver cirrhosis include:
   a) Splinter haemorrhages.
   b) Clubbing of finger-nails.
   c) Pallor of nail bed.
   d) Koilonychia.
   e) Portal hypertension.

37. Infective endocarditis can cause the following:
   a) Cerebral abscess.
   b) Erythema multiforme.
   c) Finger clubbing.
   d) Changing murmur.
   e) Splenomegaly.

38. Genuine stress incontinence:
   a) Is seen in pregnancy.
   b) Can be seen in procidentia.
   c) Can be corrected surgically.
   d) May be associated with a fistula between the urethra and vagina.
   e) Can be helped by pelvic floor exercises.

39. Features of psoriasis include:
   a) It is a premalignant condition.
   b) May be photosensitive.
   c) Can be treated with tetracycline.
   d) Lesion is itchy.
   e) Can affect scalp.

40. Torsion of the testis in boys:
a) Is an indication for contralateral orchidopexy.
b) Is less common than epididymo-orchitis.
c) Can be familial.
d) Cannot occur in normal testis.
e) Is always treated with surgery.

41. Recognized features of twin pregnancy include:
a) Hydramnios.
b) Polycythaemia.
c) Pre-eclampsic toxaemia.
d) Diabetes mellitus.
e) Elevated alpha-fetoprotein.

42. Features associated with Conn's syndrome include:
a) Hypertension.
b) Hypernatraemia.
c) Hyperkalaemia.
d) Increased renin.
e) Hyponatraemia.

43. Conditions associated with malignancies are:
a) Pernicious anaemia.
b) Dermatomyositis.
c) Psoriasis.
d) Ulcerative colitis.
e) Sarcoidosis.

44. White patches in the mouth may be seen in:
a) Iron deficiency anaemia.
b) Smoking.
c) Malignancy.
d) Alcoholism.
e) Lichen planus.

45. Characteristic features of cerebellar disease include:
a) Nystagmus.
b) Loss of position sense.
c) Scanning speech.
d) Posterior fossa bleeding.
e) Hypotonia.

46. Useful tests in sarcoidosis include:
a) Kveim test.
b) Tuberculin test.
c) Scalene node biopsy.
d) Chest X-ray.
e) Vitamin B_{12} and angiotensin-converting enzyme assay.

47. Features of carcinoid syndrome can include:
a) Bronchospasm.
b) Facial flushing with exercise.
c) Pellagra.
d) Diarrhoea.
e) Tumour in appendix.

48. The following may be seen in salicylate poisoning:
a) Tinnitus.
b) Hyperventilation.
c) Diplopia.
d) Sweating.
e) Tremors.

49. Hypokalaemia has a recognized association with the following:
a) Papillary adenoma of rectum.
b) Purgative abuse.
c) Diuretic therapy.
d) Phaeochromocytoma.
e) Cushing's syndrome.

50. In a successful renal transplantation the complications that may arise include:
   a) Lymphoma.
   b) Peptic ulceration.
   c) Avascular necrosis of head of femur.
   d) Polycythaemia.
   e) Cytomegalovirus infection.

51. The following can be seen in facial nerve palsy:
   a) Loss of taste of anterior two-thirds of tongue.
   b) Hyperacousis.
   c) Loss of facial sensation.
   d) Loss of functions of muscles of mastication.
   e) Trauma may be a cause.

52. Recognized presenting symptoms of carcinoma bronchus are:
   a) Incoordination.
   b) Paraplegia.
   c) Myasthenic syndrome.
   d) Tetany.
   e) Cushing's syndrome.

53. An apex beat at the fifth left intercostal space on the anterior axillary line can be found in:
   a) Right basal fibrosis.
   b) Right pneumothorax.
   c) Complete obstruction of left upper bronchus.
   d) Right massive pulmonary embolism.
   e) Left pleural effusion.

54. Maternal shock in the absence of heavy bleeding may be seen in:
   a) Uterine rupture.
   b) Para-vaginal haematoma.
   c) Perineal tear.
   d) Uterine inversion.
   e) Abruptio placenta.

55. **Complications associated with measles may include:**
   a) Pancreatitis.
   b) Giant cell pneumonia.
   c) Encephalitis.
   d) Myocarditis.
   e) Otitis media.

56. **Hirsutism is a recognized feature of the following conditions:**
   a) Polycystic ovarian disease.
   b) Ovarian tumour.
   c) Cortisone therapy.
   d) Turner's syndrome.
   e) Addison's disease.

57. **The following may be found in the first 6 h of cord compression at the thoracic 12 and lumber 1 level:**
   a) Absent reflexes in lower limbs.
   b) Absent sensations in lower limbs.
   c) Hypertonia.
   d) Urinary retention.
   e) Hyper-reflexia in upper limbs.

58. **The following can occur in the colon:**
   a) pH less than 5.
   b) Secretion of sodium.
   c) Absorption of water.
   d) Segmentation propels contents.
   e) Absorption of hydrogen.

59. **Stricture at a point 7.5 cm above the cardia may be seen in:**
   a) Achalasia cardia.
   b) Squamous cell carcinoma of oesophagus.
   c) Severe iron deficiency.
   d) Reflux oesophagitis.
   e) Retrosternal goitre.

60. The following may cause bradycardia:
   a) Atropine poisoning.
   b) Complete heart block.
   c) Severe anaemia.
   d) Salicylate poisoning.
   e) Adrenaline.

Paper 2   Questions

1. Consistently recognized features of testicular torsion include:
   a) Vomiting.
   b) Dysuria.
   c) Pain relieved by lifting the testes.
   d) Lower abdominal pain.
   e) Scrotal oedema.

2. Recognized features of bladder neck obstruction are:
   a) Hesitancy.
   b) Poor stream.
   c) Perineal pain.
   d) Frequency.
   e) Dysuria.

3. In the management of a boy of 5 years presenting with urinary tract infection:
   a) Aminoglycoside is given immediately.
   b) Ultrasonography can be done.
   c) Investigations are done to see if there was a previous episode of urinary tract infection.
   d) Micturating cystogram can be done.
   e) Abdominal X-ray may be helpful.

4. Unilateral middle ear effusion may be caused by:
   a) Barotrauma.
   b) Nasopharyngeal carcinoma.
   c) Sinusitis.
   d) Preauricular sinus.
   e) Wax in the external ear.

5. Retinal detachment:
   a) Is common in short-sighted people.
   b) Can be associated with sudden visual flashes.
   c) Never recurs after successful surgery.
   d) May result in unilateral visual loss.
   e) Can be a complication of diabetes mellitus.

6. Causes of pupillary dilatation during anaesthesia are:
   a) Hypercapnia.
   b) Parasympathetic blockade.
   c) Sympathetic stimulation.
   d) Cardiac arrest.
   e) Halothane.

7. Trendelenburg gait can be seen in:
   a) Congenital dislocation of the hip.
   b) Poliomyelitis which affects gluteal muscles.
   c) Neck of femur fracture.
   d) Septic destruction of head of femur.
   e) Osteoarthritis.

8. In tuberculosis of the spine:
   a) Kyphosis can be seen.
   b) Psoas muscle abscess may be the presenting feature.
   c) Early treatment includes immobilization and chemotherapy.
   d) It can be treated with surgery only.
   e) Scoliosis can be seen.

9. Hepatitis B risk is often seen in:
   a) Whole blood transfusion.
   b) Plasma transfusion.
   c) Treatment with anti-d immunoglobulin.
   d) Intravenous drug users.
   e) Staff in renal dialysis unit.

10. **A ganglion on the dorsum of the foot:**
    a) Arises from the tendon sheath.
    b) Arises from the synovial sheath.
    c) Aspiration and compression bandage should be the treatment.
    d) Contains melon seeds.
    e) Can be fluctuant on palpation.

11. **Causes of midline swelling of the neck include:**
    a) Thyroglossal cyst.
    b) Dermoid cyst.
    e) Branchial cyst.
    d) Pharyngeal pouch.
    e) Cystic hygroma.

12. **Following evacuation of a non-invasive hydatid mole:**
    a) Choriocarcinoma usually occurs in more than 20% of cases.
    b) Intrauterine contraceptive device is contra-indicated.
    c) Normal human chorionic gonadotrophin hormone levels occur in 6 weeks.
    d) Pregnancy should be avoided for 12 months.
    e) Subsequent normal pregnancy obviates the need for further HCG assay.

13. **Amenorrhoea can be associated with:**
    a) Thyrotoxicosis.
    b) Testicular feminization syndrome.
    c) Polycystic ovarian disease.
    d) Pulsatile use of gonadotrophic hormone agonist.
    e) Combined pill.

14. **Complications of surgical treatment of carcinoma of the cervix include:**
    a) Proctitis.
    b) Ureteric injury.
    c) Lymphoedema.
    d) Vaginal stenosis.
    e) Uraemia.

15. Increased frequency of micturition can occur in the following conditions:
   a) Bladder papilloma.
   b) Vesico-vaginal fistula.
   c) Utero-vaginal prolapse.
   d) Cystitis.
   e) Schistosomiasis.

16. Polycystic disease of the ovary is associated with:
   a) Adrenal hyperplasia.
   b) Decreased follicular maturation.
   c) Decreased luteinizing hormone.
   d) Increased androstenedione.
   e) Subfertility.

17. Vesico-enteric fistula may be found in:
   a) Carcinoma of the prostate.
   b) Diverticulitis.
   c) Crohn's disease.
   d) Ulcerative colitis.
   e) Ischaemic colitis.

18. Recognized features of acute cholecystitis may include:
   a) Deep palpation in left iliac fossa increases pain.
   b) Decreased air entry in base of right lung.
   c) Fluid level on abdominal X-ray in right upper quadrant.
   d) Absent bowel sounds.
   e) Increased serum amylase.

19. Conditions having a recognized association with gallstones include:
   a) Hereditary spherocytosis.
   b) Rigors.
   c) Proximal vagotomy.
   d) Pernicious anaemia.
   e) Fluctuation in intensity of jaundice.

20. Mechanisms of cause of anaemia in chronic renal failure are:
   a) Vitamin B_{12} deficiency.
   b) Folate deficiency.
   c) Decreased erythropoietin.
   d) Haemolysis.
   e) Gastrointestinal loss.

21. Plaeomorphic adenoma of the salivary gland:
   a) Never occurs in a child.
   b) Occurs only in the parotid gland.
   c) Is not radiosensitive.
   d) Can be reliably treated by enucleation.
   e) Is slow-growing in nature.

22. Recognized features of testicular torsion include:
   a) Vomiting.
   b) Dysuria.
   c) Pain relieved by lifting the testes.
   d) Lower abdominal pain.
   e) Scrotal oedema.

23. In infection with mycoplasma pneumonia:
   a) Patchy consolidation can be seen.
   b) Pleuritic pain may be a presenting feature.
   c) Purpuric rash may be found.
   d) Treatment with penicillin is helpful.
   e) Cold agglutinin can be seen.

24. The following drugs may cause peptic ulcers:
   a) Ibuprofen.
   b) Captopril.
   c) Warfarin.
   d) Alpha-interferon.
   e) Steroids.

25. Fibrinoid necrosis of arteries may be associated with:
 a) Temporal arteritis.
 b) Amyloidosis.
 c) Diabetes mellitus.
 d) Polyarteritis nodosa.
 e) Malignant hypertension.

26. Features having a recognized association with infectious mononucleosis include:
 a) Positive monospot test.
 b) Elevated IgM.
 c) Increased transaminase.
 d) Thrombocytopaenia.
 e) Neutrophil leucocytosis.

27. Incubation periods of 7–14 days are seen in the following:
 a) Measles.
 b) Hepatitis A.
 c) Diptheria.
 d) Poliomyelitis.
 e) Typhoid.

28. Brain abscesses can be caused by:
 a) Tooth extraction.
 b) Bronchiectasis.
 c) Fallot's tetralogy.
 d) Amoebic dysentery.
 e) Middle ear infection.

29. Delivery of the second twin can be done by the following:
 a) Use of the forceps.
 b) With the help of vacuum extraction.
 c) With the aid of internal podalic version.
 d) Lower segment caesarean section.
 e) Classical caesarean section.

30. Dysphagia and nasal regurgitation can be found in:
   a) Myasthenia gravis.
   b) Bulbar motor neurone disease
   c) Poliomyelitis.
   d) Oesophageal cancer.
   e) Pharangeal pouch.

31. The following may cause chronic leg ulcers:
   a) Tuberculosis.
   b) Paget's disease of the bones.
   c) Thyrotoxicosis.
   d) Heart failure.
   e) Rickets.

32. Causes of intrahepatic cholestasis include:
   a) Testosterone.
   b) Halothane.
   c) Oral contraceptive pill.
   d) Alpha-interferon.
   e) Chlorpropamide.

33. Cholestatic jaundice may be caused by:
   a) Paracetamol.
   b) Methyltestosterone.
   c) Oral contraceptive pill.
   d) Erythromycin.
   e) Chlorpromazine.

34. Features having a characteristic association with sickle cell disease include:
   a) Prematurity.
   b) Increased perinatal death.
   c) Thromboembolism.
   d) Bone infarction.
   e) Leg ulcers.

35. In face presentation:
a) Mento-posterior delivery per vagina is possible.
b) Suboccipito-bregmatic is the engaging diameter.
c) Posterior fontanelle can be felt with well flexed head.
d) Suture between parietal bones is the coronal suture.
e) Anencephaly may be an associated finding.

36. Premature rupture of membranes is associated with:
a) Placenta praevia.
b) Android pelvis.
c) Cervical incompetence.
d) Multiple pregnancy.
e) Polyhydramnios.

37. In urinary tract infections in pregnancy:
a) Right kidney is more commonly affected.
b) Vomiting may be a presenting feature.
c) Growth retardation of the fetus can occur.
d) Premature labour is an associated complication.
e) Proteinuria can be found.

38. The umbilical cord:
a) Has two veins and one artery.
b) Entanglement risk increases in twin pregnancy.
c) Is dilated in twin pregnancy.
d) Has true knots usually.
e) Prolapse is associated with frank breech presentation.

39. Hyponatraemia is associated with:
a) Cushing's disease.
b) Head trauma.
c) Diuretic treatment.
d) Chronic renal failure.
e) Addison's disease.

40. Recognized causes of stricture include:
a) Diverticular disease.
b) Bacillary dysentery.
c) Ischaemic colitis.
d) Crohn's disease.
e) Carcinoma of the colon.

41. Painless haematuria may be an associated feature in:
a) Benign prostatic hypertrophy.
b) Ureteric stones.
c) Carcinoma of the kidney.
d) Polycystic kidney.
e) Blood dyscrasias.

42. The following may be seen in long-standing mitral stenosis:
a) Left ventricular failure.
b) Diastolic thrill in tricuspid area.
c) Systolic murmur at apex.
d) Left parasternal heave.
e) Palpable first heart sound.

43. Recognized features of aortic stenosis include:
a) Black-outs.
b) Wide pulse pressure.
c) Mid-diastolic murmur at apex.
d) Left parasternal heave.
e) Systolic murmur at apex.

44. An enlarged tongue can be found in:
a) Down's syndrome.
b) Cretinism.
c) Addison's disease.
d) Amyloidosis.
e) Acromegaly.

45. Causes of pruritus include:
   a) Hodgkin's lymphoma.
   b) Addison's disease.
   c) Obstructive jaundice.
   d) Scabies.
   e) Lichen planus.

46. Massive splenomegaly can be found in:
   a) Myelomatosis.
   b) Chronic myelocytic leukaemia.
   c) Idiopathic thrombocytopenic purpura.
   d) Myelofibrosis.
   e) Metastatic tumour.

47. Recognized features of pellagra include:
   a) Diarrhoea.
   b) Confusion.
   c) Follicular hyperkeratosis.
   d) Glossitis.
   e) Angular stomatitis.

48. Sympathetic nerve lesions can cause:
   a) Partial ptosis.
   b) Sweat loss.
   c) Constricted pupils on affected side.
   d) Loss of taste on anterior two-thirds of tongue.
   e) Vasodilatation.

49. Hypothyroidism is associated with:
   a) Papillary carcinoma of the thyroid.
   b) Medullary carcinoma of the thyroid.
   c) Autoimmune thyroiditis.
   d) Adenoma of the thyroid gland.
   e) Radio-iodine therapy.

50. **Recognized features in alveolar fibrosis are:**
    a) Positive rheumatoid factor in the blood.
    b) Scleroderma.
    c) Systemic sclerosis.
    d) Polyarteritis nodosa.
    e) Ankylosing spondylosis.

51. **Scleroderma:**
    a) May cause nephrocalcinosis.
    b) Characteristically leads to deposition of calcium in the soft tissue of the hand.
    c) Can cause hypercalcaemia.
    d) Can cause hypocalcaemia.
    e) May have telangiactasis as one of the features.

52. **Vaginal candidiasis:**
    a) Is a protozoal infection.
    b) May cause pruritis of the vulva.
    c) Can be associated with diabetes mellitus.
    d) Is effectively treated with antiviral agents.
    e) Is associated with foul-smelling discharge.

53. **Obstructed labour may be due to:**
    a) Cone biopsy of the cervix.
    b) Persistent mento-anterior of the face.
    c) Mature teratoma of the ovary.
    d) Cervical polyp.
    e) Fibroids.

54. **Olfactory hallucination is recognized in:**
    a) Schizophrenia.
    b) Temporal lobe epilepsy.
    c) Atrophic rhinitis.
    d) Organic brain lesions.
    e) Petit mal epilepsy.

55. Pleomorphic adenoma:
   a) Usually develops from the deep lobe.
   b) May cause pain at the angle of the jaw.
   c) Is usually soft in consistency.
   d) In majority of cases causes facial nerve palsy.
   e) In 25% of cases is bilateral.

56. In compound fractures of the tibia:
   a) Emergency management with external fixation is the treatment of choice.
   b) Closed compartment syndrome can be an associated complication.
   c) Clawing of toes is a common complication.
   d) Damage to common peroneal nerve may occur.
   e) Hypovolaemia is a major risk.

57. Acute extra-cellular fluid loss is associated with:
   a) Hyponatraemia.
   b) Hypokalaemia.
   c) Increased secretion of arginine.
   d) Increased renal sodium loss.
   e) Hypernatraemia.

58. The following are associated:
   a) Actinomycosis and appendicitis.
   b) Tuberculosis and intestinal obstruction.
   c) Melanosis coli and purgative abuse.
   d) Aplastic anaemia and amyloidosis.
   e) Toxic-epidermo-necrolysis and staphyloccocus.

59. Increased serum amylase and abdominal pain are found with:
   a) Duodenal ulcer.
   b) Pyonephrosis.
   c) Diabetic ketoacidosis.
   d) Uraemia.
   e) Ruptured ovarian cyst.

60. Recurrent perianal abscesses are recognized in:
   a) Diverticular disease.
   b) Crohn's disease.
   c) AIDS.
   d) Ulcerative colitis.
   e) Diabetes mellitus.

Paper 3   Questions

1. **Recognized post-operative complications of nephrectomy include:**
   a) Incontinence.
   b) Hypertension.
   c) Uraemia.
   d) Pneumothorax.
   e) Infection.

2. **Regarding renal cell carcinoma:**
   a) Characteristically shows polycythaemia.
   b) Drain through renal vein to inferior vena cava.
   c) Secondary varicoceles develop in majority of cases.
   d) Secondaries to bone can be found.
   e) Hypertension is usually a presenting feature.

3. **Complications of prostatectomy include:**
   a) Bladder diverticula.
   b) Retrograde ejaculation.
   c) Impaired urinary continence.
   d) Urethral stricture.
   e) Septicaemia.

4. **Causes of swelling of the optic head are:**
   a) Retrobulbar neuritis.
   b) Respiratory failure.
   c) Increased intracranial pressure.
   d) Posterior occipital tumour.
   e) Smoking.

5. Causes of acute adrenal insufficiency include:
a) Inferior vena cava thrombosis.
b) Solitary metastatic nodule in adrenals.
c) Septicaemia.
d) Sudden withdrawal of steroid.
e) Tuberculosis.

6. Recognized features of mitral stenosis are:
a) Opening snap.
b) Mid-diastolic murmur at apex.
c) Mid-systolic apical murmur.
d) Haemoptysis.
e) Loud first heart sound.

7. Progressive cyanosis in an infant with pulmunory plethora and enlarged heart can be found in:
a) Transposition of great vessels.
b) Patent ductus arteriosus.
c) Atrial septal defect.
d) Tricuspid atresia.
e) Fallot's tetralogy.

8. Diarrhoea stained with blood is found in:
a) Ulcerative colitis.
b) Bacillary dysentery.
c) Small rectal polyps.
d) Haemorrhoids.
e) Diverticulosis.

9. Findings in rickets include:
a) Gum bleeding.
b) Low serum calcium.
c) Low serum alkaline phosphatase.
d) Low phosphate.
e) Broadened epiphysis.

10. Vitamin B$_{12}$ malabsorption can be found in:
a) Total gastrectomy.
b) Crohn's disease.
c) Ulcerative colitis.
d) Bacterial colonization of the small intestine.
e) Diverticulosis.

11. Complications of haemorrhoids include:
a) Proctitis.
b) Pruritis ani.
c) Discharge.
d) Prolapse.
e) Haemorrhage.

12. A round mass in the upper quadrant that moves downwards with inspiration may be due to:
a) Gall-bladder.
b) Liver in congestive cardiac failure.
c) Carcinoma of the transverse colon.
d) Right kidney.
e) Carcinoma of head of pancreas.

13. Predisposing factors to cancer include:
a) Threadworm infestation.
b) Irradiation.
c) Chronic lead ingestion.
d) Sunlight.
e) Smoking.

14. Erb's palsy is associated with:
a) Damage to lower root of brachial plexus.
b) Damage to muscles supplied by C5.
c) Paralysis of extensors of forearm.
d) Paralysis of deltoid.
e) Breech presentation more than cephalic presentation.

15. Recognized features of Perthes' disease are:
a) Commoner in males than females.
b) Prognosis is better in younger patients.
c) Always requires surgical treatment.
d) Presents with pain and limp.
e) May lead to osteoarthritis.

16. Trendelenburg's sign is positive in:
a) Ununited fracture of neck of femur.
b) Untreated cogenital hip dislocation.
c) Severe coxa vera.
d) Paralysis of abductors of the hip.
e) Paralysis of obturator nerve.

17. Increased gastric acid secretion is caused by:
a) Pentagastrin.
b) Secretin.
c) Histamine.
d) Omeprazole.
e) Atropine.

18. In hepatitis B disease:
a) Pale stools may be an associated feature.
b) HbsAg is positive in blood.
c) An incubation period of 3 months is found.
d) Contacted blood products are an aetiological factor.
e) Increased bilirubin may be found in the urine.

19. Causes of generalized lymphadenopathy include:
a) Primary syphilis.
b) Acquired toxoplasmosis.
c) Still's disease.
d) Infectious mononucleosis.
e) Rheumatic fever.

20. Radioisotope iodine therapy:
   a) Is associated with a high incidence of thyroid carcinoma.
   b) Usually causes peptic ulceration.
   c) Is an absolute contra-indication in pregnancy.
   d) Is treatment of choice in patients under 25.
   e) May cause hypoparathyroidism.

21. Causes of pulmonary fibrosis are:
   a) Sarcoidosis.
   b) Systemic sclerosis.
   c) Rheumatoid arthritis.
   d) Reiter's disease.
   e) Chronic bronchitis.

22. Premature labour is associated with:
   a) Cone biopsy.
   b) Fetal malformation.
   c) Uterine abnormality.
   d) Diabetes mellitus.
   e) Pre-eclampsic toxaemia.

23. Placenta praevia is characterized by:
   a) Recurrent bleeding.
   b) Lack of abdominal tenderness.
   c) Unstable lie.
   d) Previous history of retained placenta.
   e) Past history of caesarean section.

24. The following conditions may improve in pregnancy:
   a) Diabetes mellitus.
   b) Peptic ulcer.
   c) Epilepsy.
   d) Chronic pyelonephritis.
   e) Rheumatoid arthritis.

25. Innervation of the vulva includes:
   a) Genitofemoral nerve.
   b) Pudendal nerve.
   c) Anterior cutaneous nerve of the thigh.
   d) Middle haemorrhois nerve.
   e) Perineal branch of S4.

26. Phenytoin in therapeutic doses causes:
   a) Megaloblastic anaemia.
   b) Photosensitivity.
   c) Rashes.
   d) Gum hypertrophy.
   e) Osteomalacia.

27. Recognized complications of duodenal ulcer are:
   a) Perforation.
   b) Hourglass stomach.
   c) Malignancy.
   d) Duodenal stenosis.
   e) Gastro-colic fistula.

28. Causes of homonymous hemianopia include:
   a) Occipital lobe tumour.
   b) Optic tract lesion.
   c) Olfactory groove meningioma.
   d) Chromophobe tumour of pituitary.
   e) Retrobulbar neuritis.

29. Characteristic features of rheumatoid arthritis are:
   a) Heberden's nodes.
   b) Subcutaneous nodules.
   c) Pain at night.
   d) Myocardial infarction.
   e) Morning stiffness.

30. Causes of unilateral epistaxis include:
   a) Perforation of septum.
   b) Foreign body.
   c) Ethmoid carcinoma.
   d) Hereditary haemorrhagic telangiectasia.
   e) Nasal polyps.

31. Features of diabetes ketoacidosis include:
   a) Hyperventilation.
   b) Increased intra-ocular pressure.
   c) Hypokalaemia on treatment.
   d) Treatment with oral hypoglycaemic agent.
   e) Blood bicarbonate is 28 mmol/l.

32. Complications of total hysterectomy are:
   a) Rectocele.
   b) Anuria.
   c) Urinary tract infection.
   d) Hypertension.
   e) Depression.

33. Polycythaemia is recognized in:
   a) Infective endocarditis.
   b) Acute renal failure.
   c) Renal artery stenosis.
   d) Congenital heart disease.
   e) Perinephritic abscess.

34. Systolic bruit in the suprasternal notch is seen in:
   a) Pulmonary stenosis.
   b) Aortic stenosis.
   c) Coarctation of the aorta.
   d) Mitral incompetence.
   e) Aortic regurgitation.

35. Features of Parkinsonism are:
   a) Micrographia.
   b) Festinant gait.
   c) Clasp-knife rigidity.
   d) Echolalia.
   e) Oculogric crises.

36. The facial nerve:
   a) Has a sensory supply to the face.
   b) Supplies muscles of mastication.
   c) May have a sensory supply to the tongue.
   d) May get damaged in parotid gland swelling.
   e) Damage can be seen in otosclerosis.

37. Unilateral kidney swelling can be found in:
   a) Hydronephrosis.
   b) Renal artery stenosis.
   c) Amyloidosis.
   d) Renal tuberculosis.
   e) Acute glomerulonephritis.

38. Characteristic features of leptospirosis include:
   a) Jaundice.
   b) Meningitis.
   c) Conjunctivitis.
   d) Renal failure.
   e) Acute glomerulonephritis.

39. ESR more than 100 mm/h in the first hour is found in:
   a) Congestive cardiac failure.
   b) Polycythaemia rubra vera.
   c) Polymyalgia rheumatica.
   d) Polyarteritis nodosa.
   e) Cryoglobulinaemia.

40. Recognized causes of urethral discharge in men are:
a) HIV.
b) Candidiasis.
c) Gonococcal infection.
d) Chlamydia trachomatis.
e) Trichomoniasis.

41. Investigations of value in obstructive jaundice are:
a) Intravenous cholangiography.
b) PTC.
c) ERCP.
d) Ultrasound.
e) Liver biopsy.

42. Complications of asbestosis are:
a) Carcinoma bronchus.
b) Peritoneal mesothelioma.
c) Bladder carcinoma.
d) Tuberculosis.
e) Progressive fibrosis of the lungs.

43. Features of haemochromatosis are:
a) Testicular failure.
b) Oesophageal varices.
c) Increased melanin in the skin.
d) Cardiomyopathy.
e) Diabetes mellitus.

44. Causes of conduction deafness are:
a) Menière's disease.
b) Wax in external ear.
c) Otitis media.
d) Nasopharyngeal carcinoma.
e) Otosclerosis.

45. Features of squamous cell carcinoma of the oesophagus are:
   a) Commonly caused by achalasia cardia.
   b) Commonly radiosensitive.
   c) Barret's oesophagus may be a cause.
   d) Has better prognosis than adenocarcinoma.
   e) Commonest in middle one-third.

46. Causes of cataracts are:
   a) Galactosaemia.
   b) Hyperparathyroidism.
   c) Diabetes mellitus.
   d) Retinitis pigmentosa.
   e) Steroids.

47. Drugs absolutely contra-indicated in asthma are:
   a) Isosorbide dinitrate.
   b) Diamorphine.
   c) Propranolol.
   d) Doxapram.
   e) Adrenaline.

48. Characteristic side-effects of thiazide diuretics include:
   a) Increased potassium.
   b) Decreased potassium.
   c) Predisposition to gout.
   d) Digoxin toxicity.
   e) Hyperglycaemia.

49. Renal biopsy is useful in management of the following:
   a) Nephrotic syndrome in children.
   b) Hypernephroma.
   c) Polycystic disease of the kidney.
   d) Nephritis associated with systemic lupus erythematosus.
   e) Acute pyelonephritis.

50. Causes of metabolic alkalosis are:
a) Conn's syndrome.
b) Congenital pyloric stenosis.
c) Aspirin poisoning.
d) Respiratory acidosis.
e) Hypocalcaemia.

51. Features of aortic stenosis are:
a) Sudden collapse.
b) Angina.
c) Collapsing pulse.
d) Diastolic murmur.
e) Right ventricular hypertrophy.

52. The following are associated with biliary cirrhosis:
a) Skin pigmentation.
b) Commoner in males.
c) Xanthomata.
d) Pruritus before jaundice.
e) Autoantibodies.

53. Typically inguinal lymphadenopathy is seen in:
a) Carcinoma of the vagina.
b) Carcinoma of the prostate.
c) Infected calf wounds.
d) Carcinoma of the rectum.
e) Carcinoma of the anus.

54. Causes of apical mid-diastolic murmur are:
a) Rheumatic fever.
b) Aortic regurgitation.
c) Pulmonary stenosis.
d) Mitral stenosis.
e) Systemic hypertension.

55. The following are associated with unstable lie:
a) Previous caesarean section.
b) Placenta praevia.
c) Oligohydramnios.
d) Multiparity.
e) Android pelvis.

56. Features of Parkinsonism are:
a) Nystagmus.
b) Intention tremor.
c) Lead-pipe rigidity.
d) Bradykinesia.
e) Extensor plantar response.

57. Acceptable methods of shortening of first stage of labour include:
a Artificial rupture of membranes.
b) Intravenous ergometrine.
c) Oxytocin drip.
d) Ventouse extraction.
e) Prostaglandin E_2.

58. Complications of Paget's disease are:
a) Osteosarcoma.
b) Ivory osteoma.
c) Heart failure.
d) Deafness.
e) Osteoporosis.

59. The following are true of congenital dislocation of the hip:
a) Common in boys.
b) Joint ligament laxity may be a predisposing condition.
c) Commoner if one parent had it.
d) Common after twin pregnancy.
e) Common after breech delivery.

60. Causes of generalized colonic dilatation are:
   a) Purgative abuse.
   b) Ischaemic colitis.
   c) Coeliac disease.
   d) Diverticular disease.
   e) Fulminating ulcerative colitis.

Paper 4 Questions

1. **Causes of inguino-scrotal swelling which is separate from the testes are:**
   a) Inguino-scrotal hernia.
   b) Hydrocele of the cord.
   c) Filariasis.
   d) Vaginal hydrocele.
   e) Cyst of the epididymis.

2. **Features of femoral hernia are:**
   a) Often lacks pulsatile impulse even when not strangulated.
   b) Treatment by truss.
   c) Increased incidence after surgery.
   d) Commoner than inguinal hernia in female.
   e) Causes strangulation without obstruction.

3. **In third nerve palsy the following features are found:**
   a) Loss of lateral gaze.
   b) Proptosis.
   c) Pupillary dilatation.
   d) Inability to close the eyes.
   e) Nystagmus.

4. **A heart rate of 140/min is found in:**
   a) 2:1 heart block.
   b) Stokes–Adams attack.
   c) Untreated atrial flutter.
   d) Post-operative hypothyroidism.
   e) Typhoid fever.

5. Pruritus is a characteristic feature of:
   a) Psoriasis.
   b) Lichen planus.
   c) Dermatitis herpetiformis.
   d) Scabies.
   e) Polycythaemia rubra vera.

6. Conditions associated with metatarsalgia are:
   a) Pes cavus.
   b) Claw toes.
   c) Calcaneal spur.
   d) Descent of transverse arch of the foot.
   e) Ankle injury.

7. Diseases contracted from domestic animals include:
   a) Toxoplasmosis.
   b) Toxocariasis.
   c) Tricheniasis.
   d) Candidiasis.
   e) Hydatid cyst.

8. Motor neurone disease is associated with:
   a) Muscle wasting of the small muscle of the hand.
   b) Fasciculations.
   c) Ophthalmoplegia.
   d) Papilloedema.
   e) Sensory changes.

9. Prostaglandin synthetase inhibitor:
   a) Is useful for prophylaxis of pregnancy-induced hypertension.
   b) Can be used in treatment of menorrhagia.
   c) May be used in treatment of blood disorders.
   d) Is useful in management of dysmenorrhoea.
   e) May cause pulmonary hypertension in the new-born baby.

10. Causes of paralytic ileus include:
   a) Hypokalaemia.
   b) Retroperitoneal haematoma.
   c) Hypercalcaemia.
   d) Gallstones.
   e) Pancreatitis.

11. Faecal impaction:
   a) May be a cause of diarrhoea and overflow incontinence.
   b) Can cause absolute constipation.
   c) Can be relieved by an enema.
   d) Can be caused by enterobius vermicularis.
   e) Can cause intestinal obstruction.

12. Recognized features of a varicocele are:
   a) It disappears in recumbency.
   b) Commoner on the left side.
   c) Can cause subfertility.
   d) Impotence can be found.
   e) It is a premalignant condition.

13. Characteristic features of carcinoma of the kidney are:
   a) Extends through the renal vein into the inferior vena cava.
   b) Metastasizes to the bone.
   c) Polycythaemia.
   d) Obstructs the ureter.
   e) Highly radiosensitive.

14. Causes of offensive vaginal discharge in a 25-year-old female include:
   a) Gonorrhoea.
   b) *Trichomoniasis vaginalis*.
   c) *Gardenella vaginalis*.
   d) Lichen sclerosis.
   e) Foreign body.

15. Causes of generalized lymphadenopathy are:
a) Acquired toxoplasmosis.
b) Still's disease.
c) Tonsillitis.
d) Rheumatic fever.
e) Acute lymphocytic leukaemia.

16. Complications of bronchus carcinoma are:
a) Amyloidosis.
b) Cushing's syndrome.
c) Parkinsonism.
d) Peripheral neuropathy.
e) Cor pulmonale.

17. APGAR score is based on:
a) Respiratory rate.
b) Colour.
c) Heart rate.
d) Moro's reflex.
e) Muscle tone.

18. Recognized features of Dupuytren's contracture include:
a) Contraction of flexor tendon.
b) Contraction of palmar fascia.
c) Fourth and fifth fingers are commonly affected.
d) Responds to systemic steroids.
e) May affect the sole.

19. Knife stab 2 cm above the elbow resulting in inability to flex the distal interphalangeal joint of the thumb and fingers is likely to involve injury to:
a) Radial nerve.
b) Anterior interosseus nerve.
c) Posterior interosseus nerve.
d) Flexor pollicis longus.
e) Extensor pollicis longus.

20. **The following may be seen in pulmonary hypertension:**
    a) Prominent a wave.
    b) Right bundle branch block.
    c) Pulsatile liver.
    d) Increased jugular venous pressure.
    e) Loud P2.

21. **Effects of smoking in pregnancy are:**
    a) Increased incidence of abortion.
    b) Pre-eclampsic toxaemia gets worse.
    c) Low birth weight.
    d) Premature delivery.
    e) Increased perinatal mortality.

22. **Causes of osteoporosis are:**
    a) Paget's disease.
    b) Prolonged bed rest.
    c) Steroid therapy.
    d) Osteomalacia.
    e) Vitamin D deficiency.

23. **Patients on treatment for duodenal ulcer have the following associations:**
    a) Pseudomembranous colitis and antibiotic therapy.
    b) Black stools with bismuth.
    c) Magnesium trisilicate and constipation.
    d) Aggravation of chronic congestive cardiac failure with bicarbonate.
    e) Calcium carbonate and rebound acidity.

24. **Recognized features of achalasia cardia are:**
    a) Commonly in male.
    b) Aspiration pneumonia.
    c) Absent myenteric plexus.
    d) Anticholinergic drugs for treatment.
    e) Predisposed to carcinoma of the oesophagus.

25. Blood-stained discharge from the nipple can be seen in:
   a) Ductal papilloma.
   b) Breast carcinoma.
   c) Alcoholic liver.
   d) Fat necrosis.
   e) Oral contraceptive use.

26. Digoxin toxicity is known to increase in:
   a) Old age.
   b) Renal failure.
   c) Hypokalaemia.
   d) Hypothyroidism.
   e) Liver disease.

27. Diffuse pulmunory fibrosis is a recognized manifestation of the following:
   a) Rheumatoid arthritis.
   b) Busalphan.
   c) Nifedipine.
   d) Bleomycin.
   e) Nitrofurantoin.

28. Recognized features of haemophilia include:
   a) Increased incidence if mother had the same.
   b) Abnormal one-stage prothrombin time.
   c) Prolonged bleeding time.
   d) Abnormal KCCT.
   e) Haemarthrosis.

29. The following affect the nails:
   a) Psoriasis.
   b) Addison's disease.
   c) Rickets.
   d) Crohn's disease.
   e) Scabies.

30. The following predispose to post-partum haemorrhage:
   a) Twin pregnancy.
   b) Distended bladder.
   c) Halothane anaesthesia.
   d) Multiparity.
   e) Intramuscular ergometrin.

31. Grandmultiparity is associated with increased incidence of:
   a) Pre-eclampsic toxaemia.
   b) Post-partum haemorrhage.
   c) Uterine rupture.
   d) Unstable lie.
   e) Abruptio placenta.

32. Portal hypertension may be caused by:
   a) Schistosomiasis.
   b) Budd–Chiari syndrome.
   c) Coccidiomycosis.
   d) Actinomycosis.
   e) Alcoholism.

33. In acute appendicitis:
   a) Use of antibiotics removes the need of appendicectomy.
   b) Use of metronidazole has reduced incidence of post-operative wound infection.
   c) Laparoscopic techniques are technologically better than routine surgery.
   d) Two-thirds of patients spend about 7 days in hospital post-operatively.
   e) Faecal impaction can be a cause.

34. In a boy with a lesion beside the nose with fever of 39°C temperature, the following are acceptable management:
   a) Penicillin ointment.
   b) X-ray of maxillary sinus.
   c) Intravenous antibiotics.
   d) Can be allowed to continue normal schooling.
   e) Incision and drainage.

35. The following carcinomas characteristically metastasize to bone:
a) Prostate.
b) Breast.
c) Lung.
d) Colon.
e) Kidney.

36. Recommended anaesthesia to the digits include:
a) 1% lignocaine and 1:1000 adrenaline.
b) 1% lignocaine.
c) 0.5% bupivacaine and 1:1000 adrenaline.
d) 0.5% bupivacaine.
e) tourniquet.

37. Characteristic complications of a Colles' fracture are:
a) Shoulder-hand syndrome.
b) Non-union.
c) Rupture of extensor pollicis longus tendon.
d) Ulnar nerve palsy.
e) Carpal tunnel syndrome.

38. Ambiguous genitalia can be seen in the following:
a) Congenital adrenal hyperplasia.
b) Testicular feminization syndrome.
c) True hermaphrodite.
d) Pseudo-hermaphrodite.
e) Maternal androgen therapy.

39. Increased cerebrospinal fluid protein occurs in:
a) Myelomatosis.
b) Multiple sclerosis.
c) Motor neurone disease.
d) Subacute combined degeneration.
e) Diabetes mellitus.

40. The following are commoner in males than females:
a) Primary biliary cirrhosis.
b) Congenital hypertrophic pyloric stenosis.
c) Pyelonephritis.
d) Erythema nodosum.
e) Systemic lupus erythematosus.

41. Amniotic fluid embolism:
a) Is commoner in multiparas.
b) Causes DIC.
c) Characteristically occurs before delivery.
d) Is preceded by deep vein thrombosis of the calf characteristically.
e) Characteristically occurs with intact membranes.

42. The following can be used to distinguish between primary and secondary polycythaemia.
a) Platelet count.
b) RBC mass.
c) Arterial oxygen saturation.
d) Erythropoietin.
e) Splenomegaly.

43. Recognized associations exist between:
a) Polycythaemia and asphyxia.
b) Rheumatoid arthritis and amyloidosis.
c) Hepatitis and pneumonia.
d) Leukocytosis and pancreatitis.
e) Reticulocytosis and duodenal ulcer.

44. Side-effects of diuretics are:
a) Hyperglycaemia.
b) Hypernatraemia.
c) Hypercalcaemia.
d) Hypokalaemia.
e) Gout.

45. Features of chronic renal failure are:
a) Pericarditis.
b) Nocturia.
c) Increased appetite.
d) Easy bruising.
e) Macrocytosis.

46. Causes of continuous murmur are:
a) Patent ductus arteriosus.
b) Arterio-venous malformation.
c) ASD.
d) VSD.
e) Aortic stenosis.

47. Recognized features associated with an anencephalic fetus are:
a) Shoulder dystocia.
b) Prolonged labour.
c) Fetal adrenal hypoplasia.
d) Polyhydramnios.
e) Commoner in female.

48. In elderly patients treated for hypothyroidism:
a) Thyroid extract is better than thyroxin.
b) Thyroxin is absolutely contra-indicated in angina.
c) Can precipitate heart failure.
d) Radio-iodine is useful.
e) Propranolol can be given as an adjunct treatment if cardiac ischaemia is present.

49. In chickenpox:
a) Rash is limited to the skin.
b) Incubation period is 10–20 days.
c) Rash is predominantly on the trunk.
d) Can be contracted from adult with herpes zoster.
e) May be complicated by encephalitis.

50. Giving-way of the knee indicates:
   a) Foreign body in joint.
   b) Tear of medial menisci.
   c) Popliteal cyst.
   d) Sciatic nerve injury.
   e) Fixed flexion deformity.

51. Signs of left ventricular failure are:
   a) Basal crepitation.
   b) Increased jugular venous pressure.
   c) Pulsatile liver.
   d) Pulsus alternans.
   e) Gallop rhythm.

52. Conditions having a recognized association with malignancy include:
   a) Acanthosis nigricans.
   b) Herpes zoster.
   c) Venous thrombosis.
   d) Lichen planus.
   e) Generalized pruritus.

53. *Trichomonus vaginalis*:
   a) Is transmitted by males.
   b) Is commoner in pregnancy.
   c) Severe pruritus is found.
   d) Can be diagnosed by cervical smear.
   e) Responds to metronidazole.

54. *Chlamydia trachomatis*:
   a) Is an obligate intracellular parasite.
   b) Responds to tetracycline.
   c) Can cause salpingitis.
   d) Causes non-gonococcal urethritis in males.
   e) Is commonly positive in antenatal females.

55. Hypercalcaemia is found in:
   a) Sarcoidosis.
   b) Osteomalacia.
   c) Osteoporosis.
   d) Hysterical hyperventilation.
   e) Multiple myeloma.

56. Recognized side-effects of phenothiazines include:
   a) Hypertension.
   b) Photosensitivity.
   c) Jaundice.
   d) Hirsutism.
   e) Drug-induced Parkinsonism.

57. Effects of increased growth hormone are:
   a) Galactorrhoea.
   b) Hypertension.
   c) Hyperglycaemia.
   d) Homonymous hemianopia.
   e) Cardiomegaly.

58. Gonadotrophin-releasing hormone:
   a) Is a steroid.
   b) Is produced in the posterior pituitary gland.
   c) Long-term use may lead to osteoporosis.
   d) Is used in the treatment of endometriosis.
   e) Causes masculinization.

59. A cannon a wave:
   a) Is a modified v wave.
   b) Occurs occasionally in atrial fibrillation.
   c) Occurs in complete heart block.
   d) Is associated with increased jugular venous pressure.
   e) Occurs in junctional rhythm.

60. Recognized causes of parotid gland swelling are the following:
   a) Dehydration.
   b) Alcoholism.
   c) Mumps.
   d) Infectious mononucleosis.
   e) Sjögren's syndrome.

Paper 5 Questions

1. Gallstones are found in:
a) Terminal ileal resection.
b) Use of oral contraceptive pill.
c) Home parenteral nutrition.
d) Microspherocytosis.
e) Haemolytic anaemia.

2. Concerning the puerperium:
a) Ovulation does not occur during lactation.
b) Must not have intercourse during first 6 weeks.
c) Uterus involutes at 4 days.
d) Heparin is contra-indicated in lactation.
e) Lochia rubra remains for 8 days.

3. Carcinoma of the pancreas:
a) Is usually treated with resection and stent.
b) Can be diagnosed by increased serum amylase.
c) Is associated with leucocytosis.
d) Has 50% 5-year survival after treatment.
e) Is associated with gallstones.

4. Absent ankle jerk is found in:
a) Poliomyelitis.
b) Hypothyroidism.
c) Subacute combined degeneration.
d) Lower motor neurone lesion.
e) Spastic hemiplegia.

5. **Acute conjunctivitis:**
   a) Maximum infection is found around iris.
   b) Characteristically occurs with discharge.
   c) Is associated with mild grittiness.
   d) May lead to severe photophobia.
   e) Can be associated with pain in the eye.

6. **Surgery done in hypospadias includes:**
   a) Meatotomy.
   b) Urethroplasty.
   c) Circumcision.
   d) Cystostomy.
   e) Urethrostomy.

7. **Complications of massive blood transfusion are:**
   a) Hypothermia.
   b) Hypokalaemia.
   c) Hypercalcaemia.
   d) DIC.
   e) Thrombocytopaenia.

8. **Major causes of perinatal mortality are:**
   a) Hydrocephalus.
   b) Infection.
   c) Rhesus isoimmunization.
   d) Prematurity.
   e) Congenital heart disease.

9. **Recognized complications of diabetes mellitus are:**
   a) Erectile impotence.
   b) Proliferative retinopathy.
   c) Deafness.
   d) Nephrotic syndrome.
   e) Peripheral neuropathy.

10. Post-vagotomy side-effects include:
   a) Diarrhoea.
   b) Constipation.
   c) Delayed release of bile.
   d) Decreased motility of splenic flexure.
   e) Decreased gastric secretion.

11. Complications of malaria in pregnancy are:
   a) Pre-term labour.
   b) Intra-uterine growth retardation.
   c) Fetal distress.
   d) Fetal congenital abnormality.
   e) Abortion.

12. Primary post-partum haemorrhage is associated with:
   a) Prolonged labour.
   b) Placenta praevia.
   c) Twins.
   d) Diabetes mellitus.
   e) Multiparity.

13. Causes of hyperemesis in early pregnancy are:
   a) Multiple pregnancy.
   b) Hydatidiform mole.
   c) Pyelonephritis.
   d) Diabetes mellitus.
   e) Urinary tract infection.

14. Indications for splenectomy are:
   a) Idiopathic thrombocytopenic purpura.
   b) Autoimmune haemolytic anaemia.
   c) Hereditary spherocytosis.
   d) Amyloidosis.
   e) Trauma.

15. In polymyalgia rheumatica:
   a) Steroids are useful.
   b) Rheumatoid factor is positive.
   c) Age is around 45 years.
   d) Biopsy of temporal artery is diagnostic.
   e) ESR is raised.

16. Recognized features of a Colles' fracture are:
   a) Radial shortening.
   b) Extends into wrist joint.
   c) Distruption of inferior radio-ulnar joint.
   d) Dorsal angulation.
   e) Pronation.

17. Recognized causes of abdominal pain are:
   a) Diabetic ketoacidosis.
   b) Motor neurone disease.
   c) Syringomyelia.
   d) Torsion of ovarian cyst.
   e) Appendicitis.

18. Ureteric calculus may be associated with:
   a) Fixed loin pain.
   b) Referred pain to one testicle.
   c) Radiopacity.
   d) Hydronephrosis.
   e) Hypercalcaemia.

19. Causes of menorrhagia are:
   a) Chronic salpingo-oophoritis.
   b) Endometritis.
   c) Diabetes mellitus.
   d) Uterine fibroids.
   e) Pelvic inflammatory disease.

20. Recognized biochemical features in pyloric stenosis are:
a) Sodium 148 mmol/l.
b) Potassium 6 mmol/l.
c) Blood urea 18 mmol/l.
d) Bicarbonate 40 mmol/l.
e) Calcium 3.2 mmol/l.

21. Hypoparathyroidism is associated with:
a) Osteitis fibrosa cystica.
b) Abnormal behaviour.
c) Chvostek's sign.
d) Raised serum calcium.
e) Adrenal calcification.

22. Recognized complications of otitis media are:
a) Subdural effusion.
b) Seventh cranial nerve palsy.
c) Retropharyngeal abscess.
d) Cavernous sinus thrombosis.
e) Intracranial abscess.

23. In endometriosis:
a) Ovaries are commonest site of implantation.
b) Cyproterone acetate is treatment of choice.
c) Subfertility can be found.
d) Menorrhagia may be found.
e) Tender blue cysts are characteristic.

24. Primary malignant ovarian tumours are:
a) Krukenberg tumour.
b) Luteoma.
c) Granulosa cell tumour.
d) Endodermal sinus tumour.
e) Arrhenoblastoma.

25. Causes of hair loss on the trunk are:
   a) Sheehan's syndrome.
   b) Hypothyroidism.
   c) Haemochromatosis.
   d) Anorexia nervosa.
   e) Primary hypopituitarism.

26. Almost midline cervical swellings without movement upwards on deglutition are:
   a) Dermoid cyst.
   b) Thyroglossal cyst.
   c) Cervical lymph node.
   d) Ranula.
   e) Pharyngeal pouch.

27. Characteristic features of rectal carcinoma are:
   a) Constipation.
   b) Bleeding per rectum.
   c) Spread to external iliac lymph node.
   d) Pain.
   e) Response to radiotherapy.

28. Hallux rigidus:
   a) Is associated with flat feet.
   b) Can cause pain on walking.
   c) Osteoarthritis may be a complication.
   d) Interdigital neuroma is a causative agent.
   e) Can be treated with surgery.

29. Colo-vesical fistula is seen in:
   a) Ulcerative colitis.
   b) Crohn's disease.
   c) Bladder diverticulosis.
   d) Ischaemic colitis.
   e) Exposure to radiation.

30. Characteristic features of a cerebellar lesion include:
 a) Dysphonia.
 b) Hypotonia.
 c) Absent reflexes.
 d) High stepping gait.
 e) Vertigo.

31. Causes of absent ankle and knee jerk in lower limb include:
 a) Subacute combined degeneration of cord.
 b) Spinal compression.
 c) Motor neurone disease.
 d) Syringomyelia.
 e) Lead poisoning.

32. In the management of acute severe asthma:
 a) Morphine is given to allay anxiety.
 b) Night sedation is contra-indicated.
 c) High dose oxygen abolishes sensitivity of the respiratory centre to carbon dioxide.
 d) IPPV.
 e) Pneumothorax is a complication of artificial ventilation.

33. Staphylococcal pneumonia may cause:
 a) Lung abscess.
 b) Lobar consolidation.
 c) Renal failure.
 d) Hepatic abscess.
 e) Brain abscess.

34. The dose of the following should be considerably reduced in renal failure:
 a) Cephalosporin.
 b) Erythromycin.
 c) Amphotericin.
 d) Fusidic acid.
 e) Digitoxin.

35. Disseminated intravascular coagulation can be seen in pregnancy in the following:
   a) Hydatidiform mole.
   b) Amniotic fluid embolism.
   c) Placenta praevia.
   d) Pre-eclampsic toxaemia.
   e) Septicaemia.

36. Late deceleration is seen in:
   a) Cord compression.
   b) Pressure on fetal head.
   c) Cephalo-pelvic disproportion.
   d) Utero-placental insufficiency.
   e) Pre-eclampsia.

37. *Cytomegalovirus* infection in pregnancy:
   a) May be asymptomatic.
   b) Can present as an infectious mononucleosis-like illness.
   c) May lead to severe sensory neural deafness in baby.
   d) Is usually transmitted by milk.
   e) Can cause congenital malformations.

38. Precipitating factors for candidiasis of the vagina are:
   a) Adreno-cortical steroids.
   b) Antibiotics.
   c) Intrauterine contraceptive device.
   d) Pregnancy.
   e) Diabetes mellitus.

39. Recognized complications of tuberculosis of the thoracic spine include:
   a) Kyphosis.
   b) Sinus formation.
   c) Urinary retention.
   d) Paraplegia.
   e) Scoliosis.

40. Pseudopancreatic cyst is associated with:
a) Occurrence following an attack of acute pancreatitis.
b) Collection of fluid in lesser sac.
c) Pancreatic trauma.
d) Acute mesenteric thrombosis.
e) External drainage as treatment of choice.

41. The following are causes of increased secretion of acid:
a) Smoking.
b) Coffee drinking.
c) Alcoholism.
d) Secretin.
e) Acetylcholine.

42. Osteogenic sarcoma characteristically:
a) Occurs at metaphysis.
b) Has highest incidence in second and third decade of life.
c) Responds to radiotherapy.
d) Causes liver metastasis.
e) Has association with Paget's disease.

43. The following are viral diseases:
a) Encephalitis lethargica.
b) Rabies.
c) Toxoplasmosis.
d) Botulism.
e) Lymphogranuloma venereum.

44. Causes of anaemia which fail to respond to oral iron therapy include:
a) Continuing blood loss.
b) Sideroblastic anaemia.
c) Thalassaemia major.
d) Achlorhydria.
e) Chronic pancreatitis.

45. Elevation of the ST segment in V1–V6 occurs in:
a) Inferior myocardial infarction.
b) Pericarditis.
c) Cardiac aneurysm.
d) Digoxin toxicity.
e) Left ventricular hypertrophy.

46. Causes of increased proteins with minimal cell count are:
a) Idiopathic polyneuropathy.
b) Cord compression.
c) Tuberculous meningitis.
d) Pyogenic meningitis.
e) Viral meningitis.

47. The following occur in complete third nerve palsy:
a) Convergent squint.
b) Ptosis.
c) Miosis.
d) Paralysis of accommodation.
e) Diplopia.

48. Immediate indications for coronary bypass surgery or coronary angioplasty are:
a) Patient not compliant to medical treatment.
b) Crescendo angina.
c) Left coronary artery disease.
d) Positive stress ECG test.
e) Triple vessel disease.

49. Typically the sacro-iliac joint is involved in:
a) Ankylosing spondylitis.
b) Reiter's disease.
c) Ulcerative colitis.
d) Rheumatoid arthritis.
e) Psoriatic arthritis.

50. In insulin-dependent diabetes mellitus the following are seen:
a) Diabetic retinopathy is precipitated by sudden glucose control.
b) Short-acting insulin is taken just before starting meals.
c) Lipoatrophy with highly purified insulin injections.
d) Fructosaminel measures levels over past 3 months.
e) HbS prevents detection of glycosylated haemoglobin.

51. An incubation period of 7–21 days is seen in:
a) Poliomyelitis.
b) Tuberculosis.
c) HIV.
d) Syphilis.
e) HBV.

52. Tumours secreting oestrogen are:
a) Serous cyst adenoma.
b) Thecoma.
c) Granulosa cell tumour.
d) Arrhenoblastoma.
e) Dysgerminoma.

53. Causes of gynoecomastia are:
a) Klinefelter's syndrome.
b) Gastric carcinoma.
c) Spironolactone therapy.
d) Testicular tumour.
e) Cirrhosis.

54. Complications of Paget's disease of bone include:
a) Pathological fracture.
b) Osteosarcoma.
c) Chondrosarcoma.
d) Cardiac failure.
e) Optic atrophy.

55. Complications of cigarette smoking are:
a) Myocardial infarction.
b) Loss of vision.
c) Papilloedema.
d) Bronchus carcinoma.
e) Hypofibrinogenaemia.

56. Management of a 50-year-old woman with increased menstrual blood loss includes:
a) Hysterectomy.
b) Endometrial curettage.
c) Iron replacement.
d) Hormonal replacement therapy.
e) Vitamin B_{12} and folic acid therapy.

57. Unstable lie at term:
a) Requires admission.
b) Is not hazardous in the multiparous.
c) Has association with placenta praevia.
d) May occur in contracted pelvis.
e) Can occur in bicornuate uterus.

58. A neonate born before 32 weeks is more liable to die compared to those born after 32 weeks due to:
a) Incoordinated muscle action.
b) Temperature incoordination.
c) Feeding difficulty.
d) Faulty organogenesis.
e) Respiratory distress.

59. Recognized features of acute renal failure include:
a) Hypokalaemia.
b) Hyponatraemia.
c) Hypocalcaemia.
d) Polycyathaemia.
e) Hyperventilation.

60. Characteristic features of fracture of the shaft of the femur include:
   a) Fat embolism.
   b) Hypovolaemia.
   c) Compartment syndrome.
   d) Reduction is best treatment.
   e) Sciatic nerve damage is common.

Paper 6   Questions

1. Characteristic features of endometriosis include:
   a) Chocolate cyst of ovary.
   b) Subfertility.
   c) Blue nodules on the peritoneal surface.
   d) Primary dysmenorrhoea.
   e) Pelvic inflammatory disease-like symptoms.

2. Post-partum haemorrhage is predisposed by the following:
   a) Multiple pregnancy.
   b) Prolonged labour.
   c) Abruptio placenta.
   d) Cervical laceration.
   e) Precipitate labour.

3. Hypopituitarism is associated with the following:
   a) Hypothyroidism.
   b) Obesity.
   c) Increased pigmentation.
   d) Loss of axillary hair.
   e) Short stature.

4. Recognized causes of erythema nodosum are:
   a) Primary tuberculosis.
   b) Streptococcal infection.
   c) Syphilis.
   d) Sarcoidosis.
   e) Sulphonamide drugs.

5. Underlying features recognized in massive pleural effusion include:
   a) Decreased air entry.
   b) Dullness to percussion.
   c) Shift of mediastinum.
   d) Bronchial breathing.
   e) Increased vocal resonance.

6. Features of pneumonia may include the following:
   a) Normal $Paco_2$.
   b) Mediastinal shift.
   c) Increased vocal resonance.
   d) Increased whispering pectoriloquy.
   e) Consolidation.

7. *Trichomonas vaginalis* infection in a child may present as:
   a) White creamy vaginal discharge.
   b) Bubbly discharge.
   c) Vulval laceration.
   d) Erythematous rash on the buttocks.
   e) Pruritus vulvae.

8. Characteristic features of rickets are:
   a) Osteoporosis.
   b) Increased alkaline phosphatase.
   c) Widening of costochondral junction.
   d) Hypercalcaemia.
   e) Harrison's sulcus.

9. In a Colles' fracture:
   a) Above-elbow cast is applied.
   b) Distal fragment impaction can occur.
   c) Distal fragment is anteriorly displaced characteristically.
   d) Carpal tunnel syndrome is an associated complication.
   e) Avulsion of styloid process of the ulna may also occur.

10. **Patellar dislocation:**
    a) Is common in females.
    b) May become prone to recurrent dislocation.
    c) Is usually treated by cast from groin to toe with 20° flexion at the knee for 6 weeks.
    d) Is common in the under-14 age group.
    e) In majority of cases is caused by blow to lateral aspect of knee.

11. **Dysfunctional uterine bleeding is found in:**
    a) Anorexia nervosa.
    b) Stress.
    c) Endometrial carcinoma.
    d) Hypothalamo-pituitary disorder.
    e) Endometrial hyperplasia.

12. **Causes of pruritus vulvae include:**
    a) *Trichomonas vaginalis.*
    b) Candidiasis.
    c) Vulval dystrophy.
    d) Utero-vaginal prolapse.
    e) *Gardenella vaginalis.*

13. **Central venous pressure:**
    a) Is a measure of right atrial pressure.
    b) Is same as atmospheric pressure.
    c) May be raised in heart failure.
    d) May be raised in peritonitis.
    e) Characteristically raised in haemorrhage.

14. **Recognized features of Meig's syndrome include:**
    a) May occur in Brenner tumour.
    b) Is associated with fibroma of more than 10 cm.
    c) Commonly causes left-sided pleural effusion.
    d) Pleural effusion is from the abdomen.
    e) Ascites.

15. Increased frequency of micturition is recognized in:
a) Utero-vaginal prolapse.
b) Diabetes mellitus.
c) Tuberculous cystitis.
d) Utero-vaginal fistula.
e) Urinary tract infection.

16. Bartholin's cyst:
a) Is usually unilateral.
b) Originates from remnant of Müllerian duct.
c) May recur after surgery.
d) Main treatment includes permanent drainage by marsupialization.
e) Is commonly caused by sexually transmitted disease.

17. Alpha-fetoprotein may be found in:
a) Choriocarcinoma.
b) Hepatoma.
c) Renal cell carcinoma.
d) Testicular teratoma.
e) Polyhydramnios.

18. Features of pancreatitis include:
a) Hypercalcaemia.
b) Fat embolism.
c) DIC.
d) Renal failure.
e) Raised haematocrit.

19. A 15-year-old boy with a personality disorder, chorea and hepatomegaly can be due to:
a) Haemochromatosis.
b) Wilson's disease.
c) Huntington's chorea.
d) Liver cirrhosis.
e) Sydenham's chorea.

20. Contra-indications to epidural anaesthesia are:
- a) Anticoagulant therapy.
- b) Multiple sclerosis.
- c) Previous caesarean section.
- d) Forceps delivery.
- e) Local sepsis of skin.

21. Acute gouty arthritis:
- a) May be treated with indomethacin.
- b) Can be precipitated by surgery.
- c) Can be precipitated by starvation.
- d) Can be caused by diuretic therapy.
- e) Can occur with normal serum uric acid.

22. Gonorrhoea in females effects:
- a) Vagina.
- b) Cervix.
- c) Bartholin's gland.
- d) Urethra.
- e) Rectum.

23. Transverse lie at term is found in:
- a) Multiple pregnancy.
- b) Placenta praevia.
- c) Bicornuate uterus.
- d) Cephalo-pelvic disproportion.
- e) Oligohydramnios.

24. Criteria for Bishop's score are:
- a) Cervical effacement.
- b) Engagement on fetal head.
- c) Rupture of membranes.
- d) Consistency of cervix.
- e) Cervical dilatation.

25. Face presentation:
a) Is recognized in cephalo-pelvic disproportion.
b) Can be found in anencephaly.
c) Mostly occurs by chance as the head extends during engagement.
d) Usually associated with multiple pregnancy.
e) May be found in uterine tumour.

26. Recognized features of placental separation include:
a) Rise in the fundal height of the uterus.
b) Lengthening of the cord.
c) Delay in circumvallate placenta.
d) Gush of blood.
e) Uterus becomes globular.

27. Ulcerative colitis is associated with:
a) Ankylosing spondylitis.
b) Monoarticular joint involvement.
c) Gastro-colic fistula.
d) Fistula and fissures.
e) Colonic carcinoma.

28. Conditions having an association with acoustic neuroma are:
a) Phaeochromocytoma.
b) Tinnitus.
c) Sensory neural deafness.
d) Conductive deafness.
e) MEN-II syndrome.

29. Complications of Weil's disease are:
a) Optic neuritis.
b) Encephalitis.
c) Liver cirrhosis.
d) Acute renal failure.
e) Hepatitis.

30. Recognized causes of Raynaud's phenomenon are:
a) Arterosclerosis.
b) Cervical spondylosis.
c) Waldenstrom's macroglobulinaemia.
d) Cervical rib.
e) Scleroderma.

31. Recognized features of acromegaly include:
a) Increased alkaline phosphatase.
b) Glycosuria.
c) Homonymous hemianopia.
d) Macroglossia.
e) Hypertension.

32. Unilateral deafness can be found in:
a) Otitis media.
b) Sinusitis.
c) Acoustic neuroma.
d) Wax in external ear.
e) Otosclerosis.

33. The following are true of digoxin therapy:
a) It is metabolized in the liver.
b) Jaundice may occur.
c) ST elevation can be seen.
d) Used for treatment of ventricular tachycardia.
e) Helpful in treatment of hypertrophic obstructive cardiomyopathy.

34. In lesions of the large bowel compared to the small bowel:
a) There is more abdominal distension.
b) There is more vomiting.
c) Has higher incidence of obstruction.
d) Shows air fluid level at centre of abdomen.
e) Volvulae conniventes are usually seen.

35. Dupuytren's contracture:
a) Is common in males.
b) Can be treated by splinting.
c) Can cause contracture of palmar aponeurosis.
d) May be associated with diabetes mellitus.
e) May be caused by anticonvulsants.

36. Indications for exploring a patient with a head injury are:
a) Fixed dilated pupil on one side.
b) Epilepsy.
c) Pyrexia.
d) Slowing of the pulse rate.
e) Fall in the level of consciousness.

37. The main uterine supports are:
a) Uterosacral ligament.
b) Broad ligament.
c) Sacrosciatic ligament.
d) Round ligament.
e) Cardinal ligament.

38. In haemophilia abnormal tests include:
a) Increased prothombin time.
b) Increased coagulation time.
c) Positive Hess test.
d) Positive red blood cell fragility test.
e) Reduced platelet count.

39. Conditions having a recognized association with gallstones are:
a) Carcinoma of ampulla of Vater.
b) Primary biliary cirrhosis.
c) Intestinal obstruction.
d) Hypercholesterolaemia.
e) Pancreatitis.

40. Peripheral neuropathy is a recognized feature of:
   a) Nitrofurantoin therapy.
   b) Chronic renal failure.
   c) Bronchial carcinoma.
   d) Hypercalcaemia.
   e) Discoid lupus erythematosus.

41. In long-standing mitral stenosis the following can be found:
   a) Diastolic thrill at the tricuspid area.
   b) Systolic thrill at the apex.
   c) Palpable P2 at the pulmunory area.
   d) Left parasternal heave.
   e) Basal crepitation.

42. Elevation of jugular venous pressure is seen in:
   a) Superior vena cava obstruction.
   b) Bronchial asthma.
   c) Thyrotoxicosis.
   d) Congestive cardiac failure.
   e) Polycythaemia rubra vera.

43. EEG findings are characteristic in the following:
   a) Temporal lobe epilepsy.
   b) Petit mal epilepsy.
   c) Trigeminal neuralgia.
   d) Migraine.
   e) Hemiplagia.

44. The following can be causes of post-partum haemorrhage:
   a) Retained products of conception.
   b) Prolonged labour.
   c) Uterine rupture.
   d) Multiparity.
   e) Episiotomy.

45. Ptosis may be a presenting feature in the following:
   a) Tabes dorsalis.
   b) Hemiplegia.
   c) Lower motor neurone facial palsy.
   d) Damage to sympathetic chain in the neck.
   e) Temporal lobe tumour.

46. The following may be seen in severe rickets:
   a) Cataract.
   b) Tetany.
   c) Fits.
   d) Bone tenderness.
   e) Renal calculi.

47. The following ECG findings are compatible with ventricular extrasystole:
   a) Normal P wave.
   b) Inverted P wave.
   c) Absent P wave.
   d) QRS more than 0.12 sec.
   e) Notched QRS complex.

48. The long-standing effects of steroid therapy may be the following:
   a) Fluid retention.
   b) Peptic ulceration.
   c) Accelerated epiphyseal fusion.
   d) Osteoporosis.
   e) Hypokalaemia.

49. Hypertension can be a recognized feature in the following:
   a) Adrenal medullary tumour.
   b) Hypernephroma.
   c) Nephroblastoma.
   d) Polycystic kidney.
   e) Polycythaemia rubra vera.

50. Failure to grow in a 1-year-old child can be due to:
   a) Coeliac disease.
   b) Meconeum ileus.
   c) Oesophageal atresia.
   d) Cleft palate.
   e) Chronic renal failure.

51. Reasonably consistent findings of massive pleural effusion on one side are:
   a) Deviation of the trachea to the opposite side.
   b) Diminished breath sounds on the side of the effusion.
   c) Absent vocal fremitus.
   d) Dullness on percussion on the side of effusion.
   e) Low-pitched bronchial breath sound.

52. Hypersecretion of acid by the stomach is found in:
   a) Fasting.
   b) Acute gastritis.
   c) Massive resection of small intestine.
   d) Increased gastrin secretion.
   e) Gastric ulcer.

53. Management of obstruction of the sigmoid colon includes:
   a) Enema to relieve obstruction.
   b) Urgent sigmoidoscopy.
   c) Injection of parasympathomimetic drug.
   d) Oral antibiotic to sterilize bowel.
   e) Resection and primary anastomosis.

54. With regard to acute pancreatitis:
   a) Gallstones may be a causative agent.
   b) Alcoholism can predispose to it.
   c) Reduced haemoglobin concentration can be seen.
   d) Reduced total white blood cell count can be seen.
   e) May cause increase in serum alkaline phosphatase.

55. A pelvic abscess:
a) Usually responds to penicillin.
b) May cause pain on defecation.
c) Can present as anaemia.
d) May cause mucosal diarrhoea.
e) Usually shows normal white blood cell count.

56. Torsion of the testes:
a) Always requires surgical treatment.
b) Can sometimes be corrected without surgery.
c) Can be associated with inguinal hernia.
d) May present as abdominal pain and vomiting.
e) Can produce symptoms gradually.

57. Investigations in a patient with painless haematuria may include:
a) Urine bacteriology.
b) Urinary catacholamine.
c) Intravenous pyelography.
d) Renal angiogram.
e) Cystoscopy.

58. Presenting features of raised intracranial tension in an unconscious patient are:
a) Increased pulse rate.
b) Increased blood pressure.
c) Generalized convulsions.
d) Cheyne–Stokes breathing.
e) Unilateral dilated pupil.

59. Causes of recurrent peptic ulceration are:
a) Hyperthyroidism.
b) Adrenal cortical hyperplasia.
c) Adrenal medullary hyperplasia.
d) Islet cell tumour.
e) Meckel's diverticulum.

60. Generalized pruritus without rashes can occur in:
   a) Polycythaemia rubra vera.
   b) Primary biliary cirrhosis.
   c) Hodgkin's disease.
   d) Chronic renal failure.
   e) Psoriasis.

Paper 7   Questions

1. **The following may be seen in acute depletion of extracellular fluid volume:**
   a) Increased urine osmolality.
   b) Increased plasma osmolality.
   c) Increased specific gravity of urine.
   d) Raised haemoglobin concentration.
   e) Decreased skin elasticity.

2. **Jaundice in the new-born 6 h after birth is seen in:**
   a) Rhesus incompatibility.
   b) Atresia of common bile duct.
   c) Meconium ileus.
   d) Physiological jaundice.
   e) ABO incompatibility.

3. **A 60-year-old obese female was admitted in a coma. The following are compatible with diabetic coma:**
   a) Blood sugar of 150 mg per cent.
   b) Serum potassium of 6.8 meq/l.
   c) Blood urea of 75 mg per cent.
   d) Base excess of 15.
   e) Blood pH of 7.5.

4. **The following can be seen in chronic lymphatic leukaemia:**
   a) Splenomegaly.
   b) Hypogammaglobulinaemia.
   c) Autoimmune haemolytic anaemia.
   d) Thrombocytosis.
   e) Herpes infection.

5. **The radiological findings in chronic bronchitis and emphysema include:**
   a) Prominent hilar shadow.
   b) Low, shallow moving hemidiaphragm.
   c) Inflated lung field.
   d) Disappearance of lung marking.
   e) Elongated mediastinum.

6. **Recurrent attacks of pneumonia are characteristically seen in:**
   a) Emphysema.
   b) Amyloid disease.
   c) Bronchiectasis.
   d) Bronchial carcinoma.
   e) Hypogammaglobulinaemia.

7. **Recognized features of bronchial carcinoma include:**
   a) Phrenic nerve palsy.
   b) Dysphagia.
   c) Low serum sodium.
   d) Brachial neuralgia.
   e) Sensory neuropathy.

8. **Renal calcinosis is associated with:**
   a) Hyperparathyroidism.
   b) Gout.
   c) Renal tubular acidosis.
   d) Milk-alkali syndrome.
   e) Chronic nephritis.

9. **Hypokalaemia is recognized in the following:**
   a) Spironolactone therapy.
   b) Cushing's syndrome.
   c) Salicylate poisoning.
   d) Purgative abuse.
   e) Conn's syndrome.

10. The following are appropriate in the treatment of hand infections:
a) Antibiotics.
b) Elevation of hand.
c) Adequate drainage.
d) Evacuation of pus if there is swelling.
e) Physiotherapy and exercise.

11. Stricture of the colon can occur in the following:
a) Ulcerative colitis.
b) Crohn's disease.
c) Carcinoma of the colon.
d) Chagas' disease.
e) Diverticulosis.

12. Vomiting in late pregnancy can be seen in:
a) Hiatus hernia.
b) Pre-eclampsic toxaemia.
c) Multiple pregnancy.
d) Hydatidiform mole.
e) Abortion.

13. Regarding sexually transmitted disease:
a) Gonorrhoea is rare in England.
b) Treatment of mother decreases risk in fetus.
c) Complement fixation test is a specific test used in sexually transmitted disease.
d) It is rare in homosexuals.
e) Treatment of choice of non-gonococcal urethritis is metronidazole.

14. Atrial fibrillation can be a complication in the following:
a) Mitral stenosis.
b) Primary hypertension.
c) Thyrotoxicosis.
d) Myocardial infarction.
e) Congenital heart disease.

15. Recognized features of oligohydramnios include:
a) Anencephaly.
b) Postmaturity.
c) Talipes in fetus.
d) Skin deficiency in fetus.
e) Torticollis.

16. Complications of iodine 131 in the fetus are:
a) Myxoedema.
b) Fetal malformation.
c) Hyperthyroidism.
d) Carcinoma of the thyroid.
e) Peptic ulcer.

17. Human chorionic gonadotrophic hormone in urine:
a) Is usually found normally in premenstrual stage.
b) Can be found at 20 weeks of pregnancy.
c) Is characteristically raised in hydatidiform mole.
d) Can be found in prepuberty.
e) May be raised post-menopausally.

18. Regarding the vulva:
a) Carcinoma of the vulva usually occurs below 50 years of age.
b) Carcinoma of the vulva is radiosensitive.
c) Leukoplakia is treated by radical vulvectomy.
d) Acute Bartholinitis is usually due to gonococcus.
e) Lymphatic drainage is via superficial inguinal lymph nodes.

19. Regarding ectopic pregnancy:
a) Laparoscopy is treatment of choice.
b) Uterus contains decidua.
c) Commonest site is ampulla.
d) Increases the risk of further ectopics.
e) Symptoms are similar to latent pelvic disease.

20. Post-partum haemorrhage is predisposed by:
   a) Multiple pregnancy.
   b) Placenta praevia.
   c) Pre-eclampsic toxaemia.
   d) Precipitate labour.
   e) Past history of post-partum haemorrhage.

21. True proteinuria in pregnancy can be found in:
   a) Chronic glomerulonephritis.
   b) Essential hypertension.
   c) Acute pyelonephritis.
   d) Placenta praevia.
   e) Diabetic nephropathy.

22. True associations include:
   a) Bronchial asthma/tenacious sputum.
   b) Pulmunory oedema/pink sputum.
   c) Suppuration/mucoviscidosis.
   d) Pneumonia/rusty sputum.
   e) Mesothelioma/silicosis.

23. Irradiation causes:
   a) Fibrosis.
   b) Squamous cell carcinoma.
   c) Pigmentation.
   d) Leucocytosis.
   e) Telangiectasis.

24. Unilateral epistaxis is recognized in:
   a) Ethmoid carcinoma.
   b) Hereditary telangiectasis.
   c) Foreign body.
   d) Diphtheria.
   e) Mitral stenosis.

25. Recognized features of gigantism are:
a) Large tongue.
b) Large feet.
c) Prognathism.
d) Glycosuria.
e) Raised alkaline phosphatase.

26. Oral candidiasis:
a) May follow antibiotic treatment.
b) Is associated with corticosteroid therapy.
c) Can be found in debilitating illness.
d) May be a presenting feature in pregnancy.
e) May cause dysphagia.

27. Features found in aortic stenosis include:
a) Angina.
b) Right ventricular hypertrophy.
c) Left ventricular hypertrophy.
d) Diastolic murmur.
e) Systolic murmur.

28. Recognized features of schizophrenia are the following:
a) Auditory hallucinations.
b) Passivity feelings.
c) Paranoid delusions.
d) Grandiose delusions.
e) Impulsive actions.

29. The following can be found in hyperparathyroidism:
a) Increased serum calcium.
b) Increased serum phosphate.
c) Osteitis fibrosa cystica.
d) Alkalosis.
e) Renal stones.

30. Features of true extradural haematoma include:
a) It is present below the skull.
b) Ipsilateral pupil dilatation can be a presenting feature.
c) Blood may be found in the cerebrospinal fluid.
d) Lucid interval can be elicited.
e) Prompt surgery is treatment of choice.

31. Premalignant lesions of the colon are:
a) Polyposis.
b) Diverticulosis.
c) Crohn's disease.
d) Ulcerative colitis.
e) Tuberculosis.

32. Treatments of paralytic ileus are:
a) Colonic wash.
b) Cholinergic drugs.
c) Paracentesis.
d) Intubation.
e) Gastric aspiration.

33. Central cyanosis is found in:
a) Fallot's tetralogy.
b) Carbon monoxide poisoning.
c) Patent ductus arteriosis.
d) Raynaud's phenomenon.
e) Atrial septal defect.

34. Uncomplicated mitral stenosis may cause:
a) Peripheral cynosis.
b) Low pulse pressure.
c) Left ventricular hypertrophy.
d) Clubbing.
e) Loud first heart sound.

35. **Ventricular failure is accompanied by:**
   a) Cold clammy hands.
   b) Low blood pressure.
   c) Increased arterial P_{CO_2}.
   d) Flapping tremor.
   e) Delirium.

36. **It is correct to say that:**
   a) Nocturnal enuresis with daytime control in a 6-year-old should be investigated by a micturating cystogram.
   b) Febrile non-renal conditions can cause proteinuria.
   c) Paracetamol syrup is a suitable analgesic and sedative for infants with a cold.
   d) Intussusception is a common cause of abdominal pain in infants.
   e) Secondary nocturnal enuresis generally has a psychological cause.

37. **Psychosexually it is correct to say that:**
   a) Men are at the peak of their sexual responsiveness and capacity at the age of 17–18 years.
   b) Masturbation is a normal stage of sexual development.
   c) Exhibitionism has the highest rate of recidivism among sexual offenders.
   d) Female homosexual behaviour is an offence under the Sexual Offenders Act 1967 unless in private between consenting adults.
   e) Premature ejaculation is not readily amenable to treatment.

38. **Leukaemia:**
   a) Occurs mainly in children.
   b) Is commoner in Down's syndrome.
   c) May present with pruritus.
   d) May present as painful priapism if it is chronic myeloid leukaemia.
   e) If acute then in the early stages it may be mistaken for aplastic anaemia.

39. Monilial vaginitis:
a) Is a fungus that grows well in an alkaline medium.
b) Is more common in pregnancy.
c) May present as intense pruritus.
d) Can follow treatment with broad spectrum antibiotic.
e) Watery discharge is a feature present in majority of cases.

40. Raised alpha-fetoprotein in liquor amnii is found in:
a) Open neural tube defect in fetus.
b) Rhesus incompatibility.
c) Intrauterine growth retardation.
d) Twin pregnancy.
e) Pre-eclampsic toxaemia.

41. Polyhydramnios is recognized in:
a) Prolonged pregnancy.
b) Circumvallate placenta.
c) Multiple pregnancy.
d) Fetal renal agenesis.
e) Oesophageal atresia.

42. Aortic stenosis is associated with:
a) Collapsing pulse.
b) Angina pectoris.
c) Basal systolic murmur.
d) Apical diastolic murmur.
e) Positive VDRL.

43. Continuous murmur is found in:
a) Atrial septal defect.
b) Patent ductus arteriosus.
c) Pulmonary hypertension.
d) Arteriovenous fistula.
e) Aortic stenosis.

44. Recognized features of cor pulmonale due to chronic bronchitis and emphysema are:
   a) Basal crepitation.
   b) A triple rhythm at the apex.
   c) Dependent oedema.
   d) Complete heart block.
   e) Pulmonary hypertension.

45. Recognized features of subacute bacterial endocarditis include:
   a) Clubbing.
   b) Erythema marginatum.
   c) Conjunctival haemorrhages.
   d) Haematuria.
   e) Polycythaemia.

46. Drugs used in massive pulmonary embolism are:
   a) Streptokinase.
   b) Vitamin K.
   c) Heparin.
   d) Aminophyllin.
   e) Adrenalin.

47. Oat cell carcinoma of the bronchus produces:
   a) ACTH.
   b) ADH.
   c) Calciferol.
   d) Parathormone.
   e) Testosterone.

48. Testicular tumours:
   a) Are nearly always malignant.
   b) Occur mainly in middle age.
   c) May present as epididymo-orchitis.
   d) If teratomas have a better prognosis than seminomas.
   e) Cause testicular sensation to be lost early in the disease.

49. Dentally it is correct to say that:
a) Non-vital or pulpless teeth are a causative factor in the development of iritis.
b) Penicillin prophylaxis for dental procedures must be taken for at least 3 days after the operation.
c) Impacted wisdom teeth may present with earache.
d) Penicillin prophylaxis for dental procedures is best started the day before the operation.
e) Infection of teeth may be associated with cervical lymphadenopathy.

50. In otosclerosis:
a) The drum is normal on otoscopic examination.
b) New spongy bone is laid down in relation to the footplate of the stapes.
c) The deafness is accelerated by pregnancy.
d) Tinnitus commonly occurs.
e) Rinne's test is more positive than negative.

51. It is correct to say that:
a) Warfarin should be stopped gradually otherwise there is an increased risk of thromboembolism.
b) Subacute atropine reduces the flow of saliva.
c) Barbiturates are more rapidly excreted if the urine is acid.
d) Heparin can cross the placenta.
e) Ergometrine can cause postural hypotension.

52. In the treatment of idiopathic Parkinsonism:
a) Elderly people get the most benefit.
b) Has little effect on tremor.
c) Rarely gives serious side-effects.
d) Maintenance dose may need to be increased as the patient ages.
e) May be combined with an anticholinergic drug to give maximum benefit.

53. Recognized side-effects of long-term corticosteroid therapy are:
a) Deep vein thrombosis.
b) A paranoid state.
c) Hypertension.
d) Hypokalaemia.
e) Osteomalacia.

54. Painless haematuria is associated with:
a) Hydronephrosis.
b) Papilloma of the bladder.
c) Hunner's ulcer.
d) Renal tuberculosis.
e) Acute nephritis.

55. The following are recognized in carcinoma of the anal canal:
a) The majority are columnar cell carcinomas.
b) It spreads via the inferior mesenteric vessel.
c) Can present as fissure.
d) Can present as fistula.
e) Inguinal lymph nodes are usually involved.

56. Inguinal lymphadenopathy is seen in:
a) Carcinoma of the prostate.
b) Infected wound in the calf.
c) Carcinoma of the rectum.
d) Carcinoma of the vagina.
e) Testicular tumour.

57. Common complications of appendicectomy include:
a) Wound infection.
b) Subphrenic abscess.
c) Abdominal fistula.
d) Pancreatitis.
e) Bleeding per rectum.

58. Hirsutism is seen in:
   a) Stein–Leventhal syndrome.
   b) Testicular feminizing syndrome.
   c) Arrhenoblastoma.
   d) Cushing's syndrome.
   e) Addison's disease.

59. The intrauterine contraceptive device can cause:
   a) Oligomenorrhoea.
   b) Increased incidence of pelvic inflammation.
   c) Perforation.
   d) Menorrhagia.
   e) Ectopic pregnancy.

60. Following are recognized features in endogenous depression:
   a) Insomnia.
   b) Dreams about death.
   c) Early morning awakening.
   d) Diurnal variation.
   e) Tiredness.

Paper 8   Questions

1. Increased serum amylase can be found in the following:
   a) Acute pancreatitis.
   b) Intestinal obstruction.
   c) Perforation.
   d) Ectopic pregnancy.
   e) Cholangitis.

2. Hepatic insufficiency can be precipitated by:
   a) Infection.
   b) Surgery.
   c) Paracentesis.
   d) General anaesthesia.
   e) Narcotics.

3. Anencephaly is associated with:
   a) Hydramnios.
   b) Dystocia.
   c) Prematurity.
   d) Post-maturity.
   e) Face presentation.

4. Acute pancreatitis may be associated with:
   a) Acute peptic ulcer.
   b) Heavy meals.
   c) Alcoholism.
   d) Hyperparathyroidism.
   e) Mumps.

5. Recognized features of mitral stenosis are:
a) Left ventricular hypertrophy.
b) Mid-diastolic murmur.
c) Haemoptysis.
d) Left atrial hypertrophy.
e) Increased pulmonary resistance.

6. Features of abscesses are:
a) Mass.
b) Erythema.
c) Tenderness.
d) Pain.
e) Loss of function.

7. Causes of Raynaud's phenomenon are:
a) Cervical rib.
b) Atherosclerosis.
c) Scleroderma.
d) Cervical spondylosis.
e) Systemic lupus erythematosus.

8. Recognized complications of antithyroid drugs include:
a) Gastrointestinal haemorrhage.
b) Leucopenia.
c) Rash.
d) Agranulocytosis.
e) Aplastic anaemia.

9. Gastric hypersecretion is common in:
a) Acute gastritis.
b) Gastric ulcer.
c) Hypergastrenaemia.
d) Chronic atrophic gastritis.
e) Duodenal ulcer.

10. Massive splenomegaly with leucopenia is common in:
 a) Liver abscess.
 b) Multiple myeloma.
 c) Kala-azar.
 d) Typhoid.
 e) Idiopathic thrombocytopenic purpura.

11. The following are true of normal labour:
 a) Fundal dominance is found.
 b) Brow presentation usually causes obstruction.
 c) Face presentation causes obstruction.
 d) First stage in primigravida is 4–6 h.
 e) Labour occurs at 37 weeks of gestation.

12. Infertility:
 a) May be associated with less than ten million sperms on count.
 b) Hysterography is useful.
 c) Tubal insufflation done before menstruation.
 d) Fern test positive before ovulation.
 e) Usually caused by oral contraceptive pill.

13. Surgical cure cannot be expected if carcinoma of the breast is associated with:
 a) Indrawing of the nipple.
 b) Fixation of tumour to the pectoral muscles.
 c) Paget's disease of the nipple.
 d) Fixed axillary lymph nodes.
 e) Carcinoma occurring in pregnancy.

14. Recognized long- and short-term complications of thyroidectomy include:
 a) Mania and hyperpyrexia.
 b) Aphonia.
 c) Stridor.
 d) Cataract.
 e) Carpopedal spasm.

15. An undescended testis:
a) Is usually associated with pituitary hypofunction.
b) Should be fixed in the scrotum operatively before the age of 7 years.
c) Is commonly easily palpable in the groin.
d) Is more likely than a normally situated testis to undergo torsion.
e) Is associated with persistence of the processus vaginalis.

16. In the treatment of prostatic carcinoma:
a) Patients on the whole respond to oestrogen therapy.
b) 100 mg of stilboestrol daily is the usual starting dose.
c) Fluid retension may limit effective oestrogen dosage.
d) Bilateral orchidectomy is indicated if oestrogen treatment cannot be undertaken.
e) Radiotherapy may relieve the pain of the bony deposits.

17. If rupture of spleen is suspected:
a) It is important to percuss carefully the left flank.
b) The absence of bruising of the abdominal wall virtually excludes the condition.
c) Observation can be safely discontinued if there has been no deterioration for 4 h.
d) Urine should always be tested for blood.
e) X-rays of abdomen are of little or no value.

18. Recognized complications of diabetes mellitus are:
a) Impotence.
b) Trophic ulcers.
c) Callosities.
d) Renal failure.
e) Carpal tunnel syndrome.

19. Hepatic coma is associated with:
a) Morphine use.
b) Gastrointestinal bleeding.
c) Increased protein intake.
d) Hypokalaemia.
e) Neomycin therapy.

20. Diseases caused by blood transfusion are:
a) Malaria.
b) Syphilis.
c) Hepatitis.
d) *Cytomegalovirus.*
e) Infectious mononucleosis.

21. Addison's disease is associated with:
a) Hypokalaemia.
b) Hyponatraemia.
c) Hyperglycaemia.
d) Hypertension.
e) Response to ACTH.

22. Tobacco smoking is associated with:
a) Myocardial infarction.
b) Carcinoma of the bronchus.
c) Blindness.
d) Subdural haematoma.
e) Tobacco amblyopia.

23. Features of insulin-induced hypoglycaemia are:
a) Hypotension.
b) Sweating.
c) Bizarre behaviour.
d) Pallor.
e) Convulsion.

24. Recognized features of an arteriovenous fistula are:
a) Increased pulse pressure.
b) Increased cardiac output.
c) Poor limb development.
d) Distal gangrene of limb.
e) Overgrowth of proximal limb.

25. Intravenous ergometrin is indicated in:
a) Overdistended uterus.
b) Prolonged labour.
c) Previous post-partum haemorrhage.
d) Precipitate labour.
e) Uterine atony.

26. Crohn's disease may be associated with:
a) Subtotal villous atrophy.
b) Iron deficiency anaemia.
c) Stricture of the jejunum.
d) Perianal fistula.
e) Precancerous condition.

27. Macrocytic anaemia may be associated with:
a) Vitamin B_{12} deficiency.
b) Total gastrectomy.
c) Ileal disease.
d) Crohn's disease.
e) Ulcerative colitis.

28. Failure to respond to iron therapy may indicate:
a) Sideroblastic anaemia.
b) Thalassaemia major.
c) Prolonged continuous bleeding.
d) Haemochromatosis.
e) Malabsorption.

29. A pulse rate of more than 140 per minute indicates:
a) Fever of 40°C.
b) Untreated atrial fibrillation.
c) Post-operative hypothyroidism.
d) Hypothyroidism.
e) Typhoid fever.

30. Investigations useful in portal hypertension are:
   a) Sigmoidoscopy.
   b) Splenic puncture.
   c) Oesophagoscopy.
   d) Barium swallow.
   e) Cholecystogram.

31. Renal involvement is seen in:
   a) Systemic lupus erythrematosus.
   b) Amyloidosis.
   c) Diabetes mellitus.
   d) Multiple sclerosis.
   e) Polyarteritis nodosa.

32. Systemic hypertension is a recognized feature of:
   a) Adrenal cortical tumour.
   b) Adrenal medullary tumour.
   c) Hypernephroma.
   d) Nephroblastoma.
   e) Coarctation of aorta.

33. Recognized features of tetany include:
   a) Increased calcium level.
   b) Hyperventilation.
   c) A recent contaminated wound.
   d) Steatorrhoea.
   e) Porphyria.

34. An ovarian tumour is malignant if it is associated with:
   a) Pain.
   b) Rapid growth.
   c) Ascites.
   d) Menorrhagia.
   e) Solid tumour.

35. The following drugs are useful in the treatment of thyrotoxicosis:
a) Potassium iodide.
b) Potassium perchlorate.
c) Methyl thiouracil.
d) Carbimazole.
e) Isoprenaline.

36. Recognized manifestations of Sheehan's syndrome include:
a) Hypothyroidism.
b) Amenorrhoea.
c) Cessation of lactation.
d) Diabetes mellitus.
e) Hyperpigmentation.

37. Nerve injury may result from:
a) Shoulder dislocation.
b) Fracture of shaft of femur.
c) Posterior dislocation of the hip.
d) Fracture of clavicle.
e) Fracture of fibular shaft.

38. Ampicillin:
a) Is given to patients with penicillin sensitivity.
b) Is a drug of choice for typhoid.
c) May produce rashes in patients with infectious mononucleosis.
d) Is effective in trichomoniasis.
e) Is useful in *Gardenella vaginalis* infection.

39. Acneform rashes occur with the use of:
a) Cortisone.
b) Androgens.
c) Insulin.
d) Iodides.
e) Thyroxine.

40. Indications of subtotal thyroidectomy include:
a) Primary thyrotoxicosis.
b) Toxic nodular goitre.
c) Simple goitre.
d) Carcinoma of the thyroid.
e) Hashimoto's thyroiditis.

41. Characteristic features of haemolytic anaemia are:
a) Jaundice.
b) Splenomegaly.
c) Gallstones.
d) G6PD deficiency.
e) Pyruvate kinase deficiency.

42. The following features may be associated with obstructive jaundice:
a) Absence of urinary urobilinogen.
b) Pale bulky stools.
c) Palpable gall-bladder.
d) Serum alkaline phosphatase more than 40 IU/l.
e) Pruritus.

43. Proteinuria of 5 g/day is recognized in:
a) Nephrotic syndrome.
b) SLE nephritis.
c) Renal artery stenosis.
d) Acute pyelonephritis.
e) Calculi.

44. Blood changes due to drugs include:
a) Decreased coagulation due to aspirin.
b) Methaemoglobulinaemia due to phenacetin.
c) Marrow aplasia with chloramphenicol.
d) Haemolytic anaemia with digoxin.
e) Polycythaemia with methyl-dopa.

45. Splenomegaly may be associated with:
   a) Subacute bacterial endocarditis.
   b) Infectious mononucleosis.
   c) Malaria.
   d) Hodgkin's disease.
   e) Still's disease.

46. Butterfly rash on the face may be found in:
   a) Systemic lupus erythematosus.
   b) Multiple myeloma.
   c) Syphilis.
   d) Erythema multiformis.
   e) Acne rosacea.

47. Recognized features of sixth nerve palsy are:
   a) Loss of lateral gaze.
   b) Diplopia.
   c) Loss of medial gaze.
   d) Convergent strabismus.
   e) Divergent strabismus.

48. Inguinal lymphadenopathy is seen in:
   a) Syphilis.
   b) Seminoma of the testis.
   c) Lymphogranuloma venerum.
   d) Carcinoma of the penis.
   e) Chancroid.

49. True associations exist between:
   a) Hyperuricaemia and gout.
   b) Multiple myeloma and immune deficiency.
   c) Multiple sclerosis and cystitis.
   d) Pancreatitis and mumps.
   e) Hyperthyroidism and calculi.

50. Tender costochondral junctions are seen in:
   a) Teitz syndrome.
   b) Scurvy.
   c) Rickets.
   d) Secondary neoplasia.
   e) Ankylosing spondylitis.

51. Raised protein in cerebrospinal fluid is seen in:
   a) Diabetes mellitus.
   b) Guillain–Barré syndrome.
   c) Neurofibroma.
   d) Multiple sclerosis.
   e) Neurosyphilis.

52. Regarding gangrene of the finger tips:
   a) May require amputation.
   b) May be due to Raynaud's phenomenon.
   c) Patient must stop using drills.
   d) Fingers may become black and slough off.
   e) There may be a requirement for pre-operative antibiotic cover.

53. In a 60-year-old man with probable gastric antrum carcinoma shown in a barium meal:
   a) Raised ESR may be found.
   b) Pentagastrin test is usually positive.
   c) Exfoliative cytology can be helpful.
   d) Endoscopy is very useful.
   e) Explorative laparotomy is needed in majority of patients.

54. Regarding Dupuytren's contracture:
   a) It is invariably associated with fascitis.
   b) Palmar fascia is usually involved.
   c) Characteristically involves abductor pollicis.
   d) Splinting may be useful.
   e) Injury to major artery is found in majority of patients.

55. Regarding subdural haematoma in a 2-month-old infant the following are true:
   a) It can be due to birth trauma.
   b) Usually requires axial survey by X-ray.
   c) It may be associated with haemophilia.
   d) It can be treated by aspiration.
   e) The prognosis depends on the extent of brain damage.

56. Apical mid-diastolic murmur is heard in:
   a) Mitral stenosis.
   b) Rheumatic fever.
   c) Rheumatoid arthritis.
   d) Aortic stenosis.
   e) Ventricular septal defect.

57. Recognized features of primary hyperparathyroidism include:
   a) Peripheral neuropathy.
   b) Depression.
   c) Peptic ulcer.
   d) Deafness.
   e) Renal failure.

58. Chronic adrenal insufficiency is usually associated with:
   a) Pigmentation of the skin.
   b) Weight gain.
   c) Hypokalaemia.
   d) Hypoglycaemia.
   e) Hypertension.

59. Hypokalaemia is often found in:
   a) Spironolactone therapy.
   b) Thiazide diuretic use.
   c) Conn's syndrome.
   d) Purgative use.
   e) Pyloric stenosis.

60. Characteristic features of insulin hypoglycaemia are:
   a) Slow onset.
   b) Sweating.
   c) Kussmaul breathing.
   d) Hypotension.
   e) Bizarre behaviour.

Paper 9   Questions

1. **Haemolytic anaemia may be associated with the following drugs:**
    a) Dapsone.
    b) Warfarin.
    c) Digoxin.
    d) Methyl-dopa.
    e) Carbimazole.

2. **Recognized causes of reticulocytosis are:**
    a) Congenital spherocytosis.
    b) Polycythaemia rubra vera.
    c) Severe bleeding.
    d) Lead poisoning.
    e) Aplastic anaemia.

3. **Bowen's disease:**
    a) Can follow chronic arsenic poisoning.
    b) Is characterized by an ulcer of the skin with bent edges.
    c) Is a persistent, slowly progressive red scaly plaque.
    d) May have localized lymphadenopathy as a feature.
    e) Is treated by extensive resection of the diseased area including draining lymph gland.

4. **Recognized features of acrodermatitis enteropathica include:**
    a) Diarrhoea is a prominent feature.
    b) Oral zinc is an effective form of treatment.
    c) Perioral and napkin area are involved.
    d) Onset is in early infancy.
    e) Gut malignancy may occur.

5. Chronic mucocutaneous candidiasis may be associated with:
   a) Thymic dysplasia.
   b) Iron deficiency.
   c) Atopic dermatitis.
   d) Hypothyroidism.
   e) Pemphigus vulgaris.

6. A hypopigmented patch on the skin may be a feature of:
   a) Tuberous sclerosis.
   b) Lepromatous leprosy.
   c) Lichen planus.
   d) Pityriasis rosea.
   e) Halo naevi.

7. Hyperpigmentation of a patchy nature may occur in:
   a) Fixed drug eruption.
   b) Use of contraceptive pill.
   c) Arsenic ingestion.
   d) Hypopituitarism.
   e) Acanthosis nigricans.

8. Pruritus is a feature of:
   a) Psoriasis.
   b) Sarcoidosis.
   c) Lichen planus.
   d) Dermatitis herpetiformis.
   e) Chronic renal failure.

9. The following are recognized in endometrial hyperplasia:
   a) Failure of ovulation may occur.
   b) Sheehan's syndrome is usually associated with it.
   c) Dysfunctional uterine bleeding may be a presentation.
   d) Increased oestrogen is usually found.
   e) Increased follicle-stimulating hormone may be found.

10. Decreased serum potassium is commonly found in:
   a) Old people using laxatives.
   b) Colonic fistulae.
   c) Gastric fistulae.
   d) Prolonged vomiting.
   e) Secondary hyperaldosteronism.

11. Scarring alopecia may occur in the following:
   a) A kerion of the scalp.
   b) Alopecia areata.
   c) Trichotillomania.
   d) Psoriasis.
   e) Localized scleroderma.

12. Pitting of the nail is a recognized feature of:
   a) Iron deficiency.
   b) Tinea of the nail.
   c) Bronchial carcinoma.
   d) Alopecia areata.
   e) Psoriasis.

13. Ataxia telangiectasia:
   a) Is caused by a single autosomal dominant gene.
   b) Is associated with recurrent infection.
   c) Growth retardation can be found.
   d) Has cerebellar ataxia as its only neurological feature.
   e) Can predispose to lymphoma in a few patients.

14. Tuberous sclerosis is characterized by:
   a) Capillary haemangiomata of the face.
   b) Adenoma sebaceum.
   c) Onycholysis.
   d) Subungual fibromata.
   e) Shagreen patch.

15. **Oral and genital lesions may coexist in:**
    a) Beçhet's syndrome.
    b) Lymphogranuloma inguinale.
    c) Erythema multiformis.
    d) Pityriasis rosea.
    e) Lichen planus.

16. **The buccal mucosa is typically involved in:**
    a) Pemphigus vulgaris.
    b) Dermatitis herpetiformis.
    c) Bullous pemphigus.
    d) Lichen planus.
    e) Apthous ulcer.

17. **The eye is involved in:**
    a) Pemphigus vulgaris.
    b) Acne rosacea.
    c) Psoriasis.
    d) Lepromatous leprosy.
    e) Beçhet's syndrome.

18. **Vesicular eruption is a recognized manifestation of:**
    a) Porphyria cutaneous tarda.
    b) Toxic epidermal necrolytica.
    c) Fixed drug eruption.
    d) Lichen planus.
    e) Psoriasis.

19. **The following diseases are sexually transmitted:**
    a) Trichomoniasis.
    b) Pediculosis pubis.
    c) Amoebiasis.
    d) Scabies.
    e) Molluscum contagiosum.

20. The following skin lesions may be associated with malignancy:
   a) Dermatomyositis.
   b) Pemphigus malignum.
   c) Tylosis.
   d) Acanthosis nigricans.
   e) Dermatitis herpetiformis.

21. Pain and redness are prominent symptoms in the following conditions:
   a) Conjunctivitis.
   b) Acute glaucoma.
   c) Subconjunctival haemorrhage.
   d) Iritis.
   e) Trigeminal neuralgia.

22. Amyloidosis may occur in:
   a) Leprosy.
   b) Bronchiectasis.
   c) Myelomatosis.
   d) Thalassaemia.
   e) Still's disease.

23. Neurotic behaviour is characterized by:
   a) A disturbed conception of reality.
   b) Complaints for which no organic cause can be found.
   c) Denial of need for help.
   d) Malingering.
   e) The feeling of panic.

24. Surgical shock:
   a) Is linked to acute severe loss of fluid.
   b) Can be caused by septicaemia.
   c) If severe may show raised venous pressure.
   d) Slow pulse can be an associated feature.
   e) Characteristically shows increased pulse pressure.

25. **The following are recognized causes of pathological fractures:**
   a) Metastatic carcinoma.
   b) Multiple myeloma.
   c) Hypothyroidism.
   d) Hyperparathyroidism.
   e) Osteoclastoma.

26. **Irritant contact dermatitis:**
   a) Is an example of delayed cell-mediated immunity.
   b) Is a common form of industrial dermatosis.
   c) Can be demonstrated and reproduced by contact testing.
   d) Occurs frequently on the hands.
   e) Is effectively treated with topical steroids.

27. **The following may be caused by staphylococcal infection:**
   a) Acne vulgaris.
   b) Impetigo contagiosa.
   c) Erysipelas.
   d) Toxic epidermo necrolytica.
   e) Erythrasma.

28. **The following may be sequelae of streptococcal infection.**
   a) Purpura.
   b) Erythema induratum.
   c) Erythema nodosum.
   d) Furunculosis.
   e) Acne vulgaris.

29. **Scabies:**
   a) May occur as a sexually transmitted disease.
   b) Is transmitted from person to person via the adult male sarcoptes mite.
   c) Can occur as a scaly widespread rash.
   d) Usually associated with around 100 adult sarcoptes mites in a patient.
   e) Characteristically manifests as itching about 3–4 days after infection.

30. The following predispose to infection with *Candida albicans*:
a) Hypothyroidism.
b) Hypoparathyroidism.
c) Treatment with steroid hormone.
d) Diabetes mellitus.
e) Pregnancy.

31. The following may be effective in the treatment of disseminated candidal infection:
a) Oral nystatin.
b) Amphotericin.
c) Griseofulvin.
d) Clotrimazole.
e) Ketoconazole.

32. Regarding tinea pedis:
a) It is usually part of a systemic infection.
b) Is sensitive to local nystatin.
c) It can be one of the causes of pompholyx.
d) It is commonly acquired in public baths.
e) It can be aggravated by hot water.

33. Tuberculosis of the skin may present as:
a) Lupus pernio.
b) Lupus vulgaris.
c) Erythema nodosum.
d) Bazin's disease.
e) Scrofuloderma.

34. Amyloidosis may be an associated complication in:
a) Tuberculosis.
b) Rheumatic fever.
c) Bronchiectasis.
d) Rheumatoid arthritis.
e) Leprosy.

35. **Lupus vulgaris:**
   a) Is due to mycobacterium tuberculosis.
   b) Is usually aggravated by sunlight.
   c) Is characteristically responsive to antimalarial drugs.
   d) Is commonly associated with a positive Wassermann reaction.
   e) Can lead to severe tissue destruction.

36. **In early lepromatous leprosy the following lesions are likely to be found:**
   a) Skin nodules.
   b) Erythematous skin lesions.
   c) Alopecia capitis.
   d) Thickened peripheral nerves.
   e) Keratitis.

37. **In a patient treated with dapsone for lepromatous leprosy for 2 years the appearance of erythematous patches usually indicates:**
   a) Erythema multiformis.
   b) Erythema nodosum.
   c) Dapsone resistance.
   d) Lupus pernio.
   e) The emergence of sarcoidosis.

38. **Herpes simplex infection:**
   a) Can be transmitted sexually only when visible clinical lesions are present on genitalia.
   b) Usually has secondary genital lesion as severe or more severe than the primary.
   c) May cause herpetic encephalitis in the infant as a result of genital infection in pregnancy.
   d) It is an RNA virus.
   e) Is aggravated by sunlight.

39. Herpes zoster:
a) Is due to infection with the herpes simplex virus.
b) Is aetiologically related to varicella.
c) May indicate presence of reticulosis.
d) May occasionally result in loss of taste sensation.
e) Is a contra-indication to systemic corticosteroid therapy.

40. Secondary syphilis:
a) Can occur about 2 months after the primary infection.
b) Characteristically causes condyloma accuminata.
c) Often involves the palms.
d) Is usually very itchy.
e) Is a cause of generalized lymphadenopathy.

41. Regarding Reiter's disease:
a) Is primarily a disease of men.
b) Conjunctivitis occurs in most patients.
c) Hyperkeratosis lesions of the palms and soles are a feature.
d) Recurrence is possible.
e) Symptoms usually resolve in about 2 weeks.

42. Recognized features of psoriasis include:
a) Violaceous quadrangular itching plaque.
b) A chronic unremitting course.
c) A distribution which includes the face.
d) Pitting of nails can occur.
e) Involvement of the terminal interphalangeal joints.

43. The following drugs are used systemically in the treatment of psoriasis:
a) 8-methoxy psoralen.
b) Systemic corticosteroid.
c) Methotrexate.
d) Chloroquine.
e) Retinoic acid derivative.

44. Psoriasis is made worse by the following:
   a) Antimalarial drugs.
   b) Antimitotic drugs.
   c) Lithium.
   d) Barbiturate.
   e) Systemic corticosteroid.

45. The lesions of lichen planus:
   a) Are characteristically itchy.
   b) Commonly involve the face.
   c) Should be looked for in areas of skin damage and scars.
   d) Affect the buccal mucosa and the nails.
   e) Usually resolve only after oral corticosteroid administration.

46. Alopecia areata:
   a) Is usually caused by a dermatophyte infection.
   b) Is characterized by scarred areas of loss of hair on the scalp.
   c) Is associated with other autoimmune diseases.
   d) Progressively involves the whole of the scalp.
   e) Dinitrochlorobenzene has been used as the treatment.

47. Hair loss evenly distributed over the whole scalp occurs in the following:
   a) Parturition.
   b) Hypothyroidism.
   c) Discoid lupus erythematosis.
   d) Prolonged corticosteroid therapy.
   e) Use of cyclophosphamide.

48. The following conditions can present in the newborn as bullous eruptions:
   a) Syphilis.
   b) Mast cell disease.
   c) Epidermolysis bullosa.
   d) Phenylketonuria.
   e) Atopic eczema.

49. In dermatitis herpetiformis:
a) The bulla is typically suprabasal.
b) Corneal ulceration is a common feature.
c) IgA deposit in the dermal papillae can be a feature.
d) A gluten-free diet is part of effective therapy.
e) Prednisolone is treatment of choice.

50. Regarding pemphigus:
a) It is characterized by flaccid bullae.
b) Mouth lesions occur late in the disease.
c) The bullae are subepidermal.
d) Vegetative lesions may occur in flexural areas.
e) Can be associated with internal malignancy.

51. The following lesions clear up spontaneously:
a) Capillary haemangioma.
b) Keratoacanthoma.
c) Pityreasis rosea.
d) Hereditary telangiectasia.
e) Mycosis fungoides.

52. The following lesions have the potential of changing into malignancy:
a) Blue naevus.
b) Pigmented mole.
c) Vitiligo.
d) Adenoma sebaceum.
e) Xeroderma pigmentosum.

53. Erythroderma:
a) May lead to hypothermia.
b) Occasionally is a skin marker of Hodgkin's disease.
c) May follow an attack of pityriasis rosea.
d) Can result in gynaecomastia.
e) Congestive cardiac failure is a complication.

54. Cerebral abscess is a complication of the following:
a) Otitis media.
b) Bronchiectasis.
c) Subacute bacterial endocarditis.
d) Complicated fracture of the skull.
e) Suppurative thrombophlebitis of paranasal sinus.

55. Subarachnoid haemorrhage:
a) Most commonly caused by rupture of berry aneurysm.
b) Intracerebral tumour can be a causative agent.
c) Severe headache is a presenting feature.
d) Papilloedema is a recognized feature.
e) Cranial nerve palsies can occur.

56. Regarding the antenatal period:
a) Engagement of head shortly before term in primigravida implies that vaginal delivery is possible.
b) Transverse lie at 38 weeks is an indicator of hospital admission.
c) Folate deficiency is the commonest cause of anaemia.
d) External version can be done between 34 and 36 weeks of pregnancy.
e) Glycosuria in pregnancy indicates diabetes mellitus.

57. The following drugs are useful in the treatment of angina:
a) Sublingual nitroglycerine.
b) Oral beta-blocker.
c) Calcium channel antagonist.
d) Oral digoxin.
e) Intravenous nitroglycerine.

58. Recognized features of complete heart block include:
a) It may be asymptomatic.
b) Pulse pressure is usually low.
c) Cannon a waves can be seen.
d) First heart sound can be of variable intensity.
e) Characteristically shows absent femoral pulse.

59. Left to right shunt:
   a) Is seen in ventricular septal defects.
   b) Pulmonary blood flow is characteristically reduced.
   c) Can be found in aortic incompetence.
   d) Compensatory polycythaemia is a recognized feature.
   e) Blood shows increased oxygen content.

60. Cardiomyopathy is associated with the following:
   a) Motor neurone disease.
   b) Alcoholism.
   c) Ulcerative colitis.
   d) SLE.
   e) Thyrotoxicosis.

Paper 10   Questions

1. Recognized features of sarcoidosis include:
   a) Clubbing of fingures.
   b) Erythema nodosum.
   c) Hilar lymphadenopathy.
   d) Positive Mantoux test.
   e) Iritis.

2. Pulmonary metastasis are characteristically seen in the following:
   a) Carcinoma of the cervix.
   b) Seminoma.
   c) Multiple myeloma.
   d) Osteosarcoma.
   e) Astrocytoma.

3. Nerve injury may occur in the following:
   a) Shoulder dislocation.
   b) Fracture of hip.
   c) Fracture of clavicle.
   d) Fracture of tibia.
   e) Fracture of ulna.

4. Recognized causes of fistulas in ano are:
   a) Crohn's disease.
   b) Ulcerative colitis.
   c) Tuberculosis.
   d) Bilharziasis.
   e) Lymphogranuloma venerum.

5. At birth:
a) Nails up to the end of the fingers are usually seen.
b) Moro's reflex is normally present.
c) Lanugo hair is seen.
d) Grasp reflex is positive.
e) Anterior fontanelle is closed.

6. Regarding secondary post-partum haemorrhage:
a) Exploration is a must.
b) Bimanual pressure is usually given.
c) It can be due to overdistension.
d) Ergometrin can be given.
e) Cervical erosion is a major cause.

7. Cervical carcinoma in situ:
a) Is histologically characteristic.
b) May not be necessarily invasive.
c) Is associated with good prognosis.
d) Simple hysterectomy is indicated as treatment.
e) Cone biopsy is sufficient.

8. Complications of intravenous pentothal sodium are:
a) Hypotension.
b) Laryngeal spasm.
c) Respiratory arrest.
d) Damage to liver.
e) Venous thrombosis.

9. Lumbar sympathectomy:
a) Increases blood flow to the skin.
b) May cause hypotension.
c) Helps in relieving pain in Buerger's disease.
d) Can cure incipient gangrene in atherosclerosis.
e) Can cause oedema of the leg.

10. **Complications of sliding hiatus hernia include:**
    a) Pernicious anaemia.
    b) Iron deficiency anaemia.
    c) Oesophageal stricture.
    d) Oesophageal varices.
    e) Chest pain.

11. **The following are recognized causes of anal pain:**
    a) Prolapsed piles.
    b) Fissure in anus.
    c) Carcinoma of the rectum.
    d) Pilonidal sinus.
    e) Ischiorectal abscess.

12. **Bulging of the anterior fontanelle in infants is seen in:**
    a) Microcephaly.
    b) Bacterial meningitis.
    c) Subdural haematoma.
    d) Dehydration.
    e) Hydrocephalus.

13. **Post-operative pulmonary collapse is seen in:**
    a) Smokers.
    b) Chronic bronchitis.
    c) History of tuberculosis.
    d) Lower abdominal incision.
    e) Pulmonary embolism.

14. **Stridor is a recognized feature in the following:**
    a) Simple goitre.
    b) Carcinoma of the thyroid.
    c) Angioneurotic oedema.
    d) Hysteria.
    e) Recurrent laryngeal nerve palsy.

15. Large bowel obstruction:
a) Can be caused by diverticulosis of the colon.
b) Is more common in the elderly.
c) Usually has vomiting as the earliest symptom.
d) May show increased bowel sound.
e) Characteristically shows with constipation and distension.

16. Extensor plantar reflex is seen in the following:
a) Infants under 6 years of age.
b) Pyramidal lesions.
c) Subacute combined degeneration.
d) Peripheral neuritis.
e) Friedreich's ataxia.

17. The following are true of acute appendicitis:
a) Anorexia may be present.
b) Aphthous ulcers are usual presentation.
c) May cause septicaemia.
d) Never occurs in elderly.
e) Usually does not occur in pregnancy.

18. The following are recognized complications in fracture of the shaft of the femur:
a) Hypovolaemia.
b) Haemarthrosis of the femur.
c) Fat embolism.
d) Gangrene of the toes.
e) Sciatic nerve injury.

19. Recognized causes of non-union in a fracture include:
a) Infection.
b) Impaired blood supply.
c) Interruption of soft tissue.
d) Overlapping of fragments.
e) Metastatic carcinoma.

20. Features seen in giant cell arteritis include:
   a) Uniocular blindness.
   b) Low ESR.
   c) Headache.
   d) Response to treatment with steroid.
   e) Cranial nerve palsy.

21. An abnormal Schilling's test is seen in:
   a) Crohn's disease.
   b) Ulcerative colitis.
   c) Total gastrectomy.
   d) Multiple jejunal diverticulosis.
   e) Pernicious anaemia.

22. Acute pancreatitis is associated with:
   a) Hypercalcaemia.
   b) Alcoholism.
   c) Increased serum amylase in 24 h.
   d) Acute renal failure.
   e) Peripheral circulatory failure.

23. Small muscle wasting is seen in the following:
   a) Motor neurone disease.
   b) Poliomyelitis.
   c) Rheumatoid arthritis.
   d) Multiple sclerosis.
   e) Carpal tunnel syndrome.

24. Glycosuria can occur in the following:
   a) Thiazide diuretic treatment.
   b) Pancreatitis.
   c) Cystic fibrosis.
   d) Conn's syndrome.
   e) Cushing's syndrome.

25. Recognized features of acute appendicitis in a 12-year-old boy include:
a) Rovsing's sign.
b) Umbilical pain.
c) More than 10 pus cells in urine.
d) Bronchial breathing.
e) Diarrhoea.

26. Features of patent ductus arteriosus include:
a) Right to left shunt.
b) Cardiomegaly.
c) Increased pulmonary resistance.
d) Cyanosis.
e) Machinery murmur.

27. With regard to claudication pain:
a) Surgery is usually required after 2 years.
b) It is commonest in the calf.
c) May occur in buttocks and thigh.
d) It is usually due to inadequate blood supply.
e) Claudication distance is affected by general health of the patient.

28. Malformation of teeth may be seen in the following:
a) Congenital syphilis.
b) Fluorosis.
c) Avitaminosis C.
d) Avitaminosis D.
e) Avitaminosis B_{12}.

29. The following have a recognized association with transverse lie:
a) Multiple pregnancy.
b) Subseptate uterus.
c) Hydramnios.
d) Contracted pelvis.
e) Oligohydramnios.

30. Hypertension may be caused by:
   a) Primary hyperaldosteronism.
   b) Pheochromocytoma.
   c) Cushing's syndrome.
   d) Addison's disease.
   e) Coarctation of aorta.

31. Aspiration is commonly seen in:
   a) Cuffed endotracheal tube.
   b) Left lateral position.
   c) Comatose patient.
   d) Ineffective post-operative cough.
   e) Laryngeal paralysis.

32. Consistent features of the leg in a fracture of the neck of the femur include:
   a) Shortening.
   b) External rotation.
   c) Internal rotation.
   d) Pain on flexion.
   e) Abduction.

33. Recognized features of portal hypertension include:
   a) Splenomegaly.
   b) Pigmentation.
   c) Ascites.
   d) Anaemia.
   e) Ankle oedema.

34. Diseases caused by viruses are:
   a) Infectious mononucleosis.
   b) Toxoplasmosis.
   c) Lymphogranuloma venerum.
   d) Measles.
   e) Mumps.

35. Extensor plantar reflex is a recognized finding in the following:
   a) Subacute combined degeneration of the cord.
   b) Lower motor lesion.
   c) Upper motor lesion.
   d) Coma.
   e) Epilepsy.

36. The following conditions are associated with haemoptysis:
   a) Pulmonary hypertension.
   b) Bronchiectasis.
   c) Mitral stenosis.
   d) Hypernephroma.
   e) Pulmonary tuberculosis.

37. Postmaturity is a recognized complication of the following:
   a) Diabetes mellitus.
   b) Pre-eclampsic toxaemia.
   c) Anencephaly.
   d) Multiple pregnancy.
   e) Hydramnios.

38. In a hyperosmolar non-ketotic diabetic coma:
   a) Blood sugar is rarely above 33.4 mmol/l.
   b) PCV is usually less than 30.
   c) Mortality is quite high.
   d) Patient is usually insulin dependent.
   e) Plasma pH is always less than 7.25.

39. The following vaccines contain live organisms:
   a) Diphtheria.
   b) Rubella.
   c) Measles.
   d) Poliomyelitis.
   e) Smallpox.

40. Dementia is a recognized sequela of the following:
a) Lead poisoning.
b) Cushing's disease.
c) Aseptic meningitis.
d) Brain neoplasm.
e) Huntington's chorea.

41. It is correct to say that:
a) In carcinoma of the distal colon increasing constipation is usually the first symptom.
b) The usual type of anaemia in the post-gastrectomy period is megaloblastic.
c) A past history of piles often delays the diagnosis of carcinoma of the rectum.
d) Diverticulosis should be treated with a low roughage diet and faecal softeners.
e) Pale stools and urobilinogen in the urine are characteristic of obstructive jaundice.

42. The following statements are true of gout:
a) It is a true arthritis.
b) It is commoner in females.
c) Increased uric acid production can be found.
d) Renal calculi may occur.
e) Deficiency of glucose-6-phosphatase is a recognized cause.

43. Pancytopenia is associated with the following:
a) Severe folic acid deficiency.
b) Chronic lymphatic leukaemia.
c) Infectious mononucleosis.
d) Aplastic anaemia.
e) SLE.

44. The following features are consistent with the diagnosis of thyrotoxicosis:
a) Proximal myopathy.
b) Peripheral neuropathy.
c) Opthalmoplegia.
d) Atrial fibrillation.
e) Tremors.

45. Recognized features of whooping cough include:
   a) Incubation period of 7–14 days.
   b) Caused by droplet infection.
   c) Convulsions.
   d) Leucopenia.
   e) Lymphocytosis.

46. Metronidazole therapy may be useful in infections of the following:
   a) Bacteroides.
   b) Clostridium.
   c) Entamoeba histolytica.
   d) Staphylococcus.
   e) Giardia lamblia.

47. The following are characteristic features of Sheehan's syndrome:
   a) Hypothyroidism.
   b) Failure of lactation.
   c) Pigmentation.
   d) Dysmenorrhoea.
   e) Loss of axillary and pubic hair.

48. Infection of an amputation stump with *Clostridium welchii*:
   a) Is associated with high fever throughout the course of the illness.
   b) Should usually be treated with penicillin.
   c) Produces a characteristic sensation on palpation of the affected part.
   d) Is an indication of hyperbaric oxygen therapy.
   e) Typically occurs several weeks after the amputation.

49. Following acute haemorrhage:
   a) Pallor and sweating are evidence of sympathetic overactivity.
   b) The patient should be kept warm to restore skin blood flow.
   c) Central venous pressure usually falls.
   d) Renal tubular necrosis is a recognized complication.
   e) The degree of hypotension is a reliable index of the amount of blood loss.

50. The immediate management of severe chest injury should include:

a) Firm support of the detached segment if a flail chest is present.
b) Bronchoscopy to exclude rupture of bronchus.
c) Drainage of a tension pneumothorax via an underwater seal if present.
d) Surgical exploration if the venous pressure is rising and the blood pressure falling.
e) An early chest X-ray.

51. A varicose ulcer:

a) May be preceded by a flare of venules over the malleollus.
b) Should be treated with local antibiotics if infection has occurred.
c) Recurs in about two-thirds of cases unless the associated varicose veins are treated effectively.
d) Can be a recognized long-term result of deep vein thrombosis.
e) Usually due to high pressure in the superficial veins.

52. In a patient who is unconscious following a head injury:

a) Tachycardia and hypotension indicate increasing cerebral compression.
b) Changes in the level of consciousness are the most important guide to the need for surgery.
c) If pupils are unequal a light shone into the dilated pupil will usually produce constriction of the opposite pupil.
d) Full recovery can be expected more often than not.
e) A period of normal consciousness following the injury is suggestive of extradural haemorrhage.

53. The following toxic effects can be seen 48h after an overdose:

a) Tinnitus with aspirin.
b) Jaundice with paracetamol.
c) Lung damage with paraquat.
d) Cardiac arrhythmias with tricyclics.
e) Agranulocytosis with phenylbutazone.

54. Recognized features of cervical spondylosis are:
a) Inflammation of cervical spine.
b) Commoner in men.
c) Intervertebral disc degeneration.
d) Osteophyte formation.
e) Biochemical changes in cerebrospinal fluid.

55. Delayed recovery following general anaesthesia can be due to:
a) Anoxic episode.
b) Carbon dioxide narcosis.
c) High dose of pre-operative narcotic.
d) Residual curarization.
e) Hyperventilation.

56. With regard to breast carcinoma:
a) Abortion should be done if pregnant within 1 year of mastectomy.
b) There is increased incidence of breast carcinoma in the opposite side.
c) It is found to be more common in unmarried women.
d) A normal X-ray excludes metastasis.
e) Palpable axillary lymph nodes indicate inoperability.

57. Early features of intussusception in infancy are:
a) Pallor.
b) Chronic constipation.
c) Abdominal distension.
d) Pain.
e) Passage of blood PR.

58. Treatment of dry gangrene of the tip of the finger in a manual worker includes:
a) Digital endarterectomy.
b) Amputation of distal phalanx.
c) Amputation of digit.
d) Administration of nicotinic acid.
e) Not to use pneumatic drills.

59. The following may be seen in pheochromocytoma:
   a) Increased urinary VMA.
   b) Increased serum catecholamines.
   c) Incresed urinary 5HIAA.
   d) Decreased GFR.
   e) Increased blood sugar.

60. Oligohydramnios is associated with the following conditions:
   a) Diabetes mellitus.
   b) Postmaturity.
   c) Rhesus incompatibility.
   d) Renal agenesis.
   e) Haemangioma of the placenta.

Paper 11   Questions

1. Mental retardation is a recognized feature in the following:
   a) Mumps.
   b) Hepatitis.
   c) Toxoplasmosis.
   d) Cytomegalovirus infection.
   e) Chicken-pox.

2. Normal uterine contraction:
   a) Usually causes increase in placental blood flow.
   b) Spreads from muscle fibre to fibre directly.
   c) Invariably originates in uterotubal junction.
   d) May cause increased intrauterine pressure.
   e) Can be reduced by oxytocin administration.

3. Incidence of post-partum haemorrhage is increased in:
   a) General anaesthesia with halothane.
   b) Maternal anaemia.
   c) Precipitate labour.
   d) Multiparity.
   e) Ante-partum haemorrhage.

4. Vaginal bleeding in the first 20 weeks of pregnancy can be due to:
   a) Ectopic pregnancy.
   b) Primary labour.
   c) Hydatidiform mole.
   d) Abruptio placenta.
   e) Carcinoma of the cervix.

5. Ectopic pregnancy can occur in the following sites:
a) Abdominal cavity.
b) Ovary.
c) Fallopian tube.
d) Cornua of uterus.
e) Cervix.

6. Carcinoma of the endometrium may be associated with:
a) Smoking.
b) Oestrogen therapy.
c) Diabetes mellitus.
d) Endometriosis.
e) Endometrial hyperplasia.

7. Dwarfism is a recognized feature in:
a) Cretinism.
b) Achondroplasia.
c) Down's syndrome.
d) Kleinfelter's syndrome.
e) Coeliac disease.

8. Thrombocytopenia has a known association with:
a) Salicylate use.
b) Hypersplenism.
c) Acute leukaemia.
d) SLE.
e) Lymphoma.

9. In chronic active hepatitis:
a) Recurrence of jaundice may be a feature.
b) Decrease in immunoglobulin usually occurs.
c) Piecemeal necrosis of the liver is a recognized complication.
d) Autoantibodies may be increased.
e) Cirrhosis of the liver may be a sequel.

10. **Measurements with prognostic value in pre-eclampsic toxaemia include:**
    a) Proteinuria.
    b) Urine output.
    c) Blood pressure.
    d) Pulse.
    e) Temperature.

11. **Immunosuppressive therapy is useful in:**
    a) Nephrotic syndrome.
    b) Proliferative glomerulonephritis.
    c) Lupus nephritis.
    d) Goodpasture's syndrome.
    e) Wegener's glomerulonephritis.

12. **The following can be found in iron deficiency anaemia:**
    a) Microcytosis.
    b) Hypochromia.
    c) Anisocytosis.
    d) Poikilocytosis.
    e) Decreased iron-binding capacity.

13. **Following a fracture or dislocation of the spine:**
    a) Permanent neurological damage is unlikely if the affected vertebra is wedged.
    b) The stability of the fracture depends on the integrity of the supraspinous ligament.
    c) Full recovery is impossible if the cauda equina is injured.
    d) Full recovery from quadriplegia can be confidently expected if the lateral X-ray of the cervical spine is normal.
    e) The early evidence of cord transection includes flaccid paralysis, retention of urine and priapism.

14. The most likely cause of dysphagia:
a) In an elderly male is carcinoma of the oesophagus.
b) Is simple stricture if there is a history of reflux oesophagitis.
c) In a young female with progressive severe weight loss is achalasia cardia.
d) Is a foreign body if there is pain on swallowing.
e) In an infant of 2 weeks is oesophageal atresia.

15. Congenital hypertrophic pyloric stenosis:
a) Is a condition of unknown aetiology.
b) Only rarely occurs in siblings.
c) Typically presents within a day or two of birth.
d) Demands a few days of pre-operative preparation in severe cases.
e) Responds as well to atropine methylnitrate as to operation.

16. Acute appendicitis:
a) Is only prevalent in people taking a western diet.
b) May occur in a non-obstructed appendix.
c) Produces pain which is referred to the right iliac fossa irrespective of the anatomical position of the appendix.
d) Gives pain which causes the patient to writhe about.
e) Has a higher mortality in pregnancy.

17. In a case of jaundice:
a) A family history of anaemia may give a clue to the diagnosis.
b) Enquiry about drugs is important.
c) A history of severe pain and rigors suggests viral hepatitis.
d) Continuous pain radiating to the back suggests malignant disease.
e) Tenderness of the liver is strongly suggestive of cirrhosis of the liver.

18. Late complications of peptic ulcer surgery are:
a) Vomiting.
b) Diarrhoea.
c) Iron deficiency anaemia.
d) Pancreatitis.
e) Postcibal syndrome.

19. Useful treatments in diabetic ketoacidosis include:
a) Rehydration.
b) Insulin.
c) Ammonium chloride by mouth.
d) Blood transfusion.
e) Oral hypoglycaemic agents.

20. Regarding breech presentation:
a) Breech extraction of dead fetus can be done.
b) It is associated with multiparas.
c) It is associated with fetal monsters.
d) It has an association with multiple pregnancy.
e) It is associated with contracted pelvis.

21. A white cell count of more than 15 000 per mm^3 is suggestive of:
a) Acute appendicitis.
b) Diphtheria.
c) Viral pneumonia.
d) Typhoid.
e) SLE.

22. Fresh blood in the stools is seen in the following:
a) Amoebiasis.
b) Ankylostoma duodenal infestation.
c) Carcinoma of the rectum.
d) Fissure in ano.
e) Haemorrhoids.

23. Hallucinations can occur in the following:
a) Delirium.
b) Manic depression.
c) Schizophrenia.
d) Obsessive neurosis.
e) Alcoholics.

24. In osteogenic sarcoma:
   a) The 5-year survival rate is 50% following adequate treatment.
   b) Block dissection of involved lymph nodes is usually helpful.
   c) The commonest mode of spread is blood-borne.
   d) Paget's disease may be an association.
   e) Excessive irradiation is one of the causes.

25. Raised intracranial pressure:
   a) May present as papilloedema.
   b) Can cause epilepsy.
   c) Can present as bitemporal hemianopia.
   d) Can be a recognized complication of meningitis.
   e) Can be caused by an intracranial tumour.

26. Benign prostatic hypertrophy can present as:
   a) Hesitancy.
   b) Increased frequency of micturition.
   c) Haematuria.
   d) Pain in tip of penis.
   e) Impotence.

27. Recognized features of pernicious anaemia include:
   a) Confusion.
   b) Epilepsy.
   c) Achlorhydria.
   d) Urobilinogen in urine.
   e) Tingling and numbness.

28. Miliary mottling in X-rays can be seen in:
   a) Sarcoidosis.
   b) Asbestosis.
   c) Toxoplasmosis.
   d) Miliary tuberculosis.
   e) Silicosis.

29. Visual loss is a known complication of use of the following drugs:
   a) Barbiturates.
   b) Ethambutol.
   c) Halothane.
   d) Oxygen.
   e) Chloroquine.

30. The following conditions may lead to hypercapnia:
   a) Chronic bronchitis.
   b) Diabetic ketoacidosis.
   c) Acute asthma.
   d) Severe barbiturate poisoning.
   e) Hysterical hyperventilation.

31. Hair loss can be found in:
   a) Psoriasis.
   b) No obvious cause.
   c) Secondary syphilis.
   d) Early diabetes mellitus.
   e) Cyclophosphamide use.

32. Which of the following may show with palmar erythema?:
   a) Pregnancy.
   b) Thyrotoxicosis.
   c) Addison's disease.
   d) Osteoarthritis.
   e) Cirrhosis of the liver.

33. Recognized features of acute glaucoma include:
   a) Decrease in visual fields.
   b) Papilloedema.
   c) Red eye.
   d) Keratitis.
   e) Frontal headache.

34. Features associated with carcinoid syndrome include:
   a) Diarrhoea.
   b) Constipation.
   c) Flushing.
   d) Liver secondaries.
   e) Severe duodenal ulcer.

35. Defects in the form of chromosomal anomalies can be found in:
   a) Down's syndrome.
   b) Achondroplasia.
   c) Turner's syndrome.
   d) Kleinfelter's syndrome.
   e) Osteogenesis imperfecta.

36. Complications of gastrectomy may include the following:
   a) Malabsorption syndrome.
   b) Macrocytic anaemia.
   c) Postcibal syndrome.
   d) Constipation.
   e) Osteomalacia.

37. Iron absorption:
   a) Is impaired after partial gastrectomy.
   b) Can be seen in adult coeliac desease.
   c) Is better at low pH of the gut.
   d) Is better at high pH of the gut.
   e) Is increased with high pancreatic secretion.

38. Characteristic features of depression include:
   a) Early morning awakening.
   b) Auditory hallucinations.
   c) Paranoid ideations.
   d) Feelings of guilt.
   e) Delusion of grandiosity.

39. Typical features of left-sided nerve deafness include:
a) Hears better on left with tuning fork on vertex.
b) Wax in external ear.
c) Air conduction better than bone conduction in left ear.
d) Air conduction better than bone conduction in right ear.
e) No conductive deafness in left ear.

40. Features in a patient with iritis include:
a) Pain is severe enough to keep the patient awake at night.
b) Photophobia can be relieved by dark glasses.
c) Pupils are dilated.
d) Pupils can be irregular.
e) Profuse conjunctival discharge can be seen.

41. Paget's disease of the nipple:
a) Is usually bilateral.
b) Is eczema of the nipple.
c) Shows specific histological appearance.
d) Treatment includes local excision of the nipple.
e) Is always associated with neoplasm of the breast.

42. Post-operative pulmonary embolism:
a) Is usually preceded by signs of deep vein thrombosis.
b) Blood-stained sputum is a recognized feature.
c) Does not occur after splenectomy.
d) May cause pleuritic pain.
e) Is usually less likely if patient is receiving prophylactic anticoagulant.

43. The following investigations are useful in painless haematuria:
a) Culture urine.
b) Urinary catecholamines.
c) Intravenous pyelography.
d) Renal angiogram.
e) Cystoscopy.

44. **Subtotal thyroidectomy as a treatment is useful in the following conditions:**
    a) Multinodular goitre.
    b) Puberty goitre.
    c) Toxic goitre.
    d) Hashimoto's thyroiditis.
    e) Subacute thyroiditis.

45. **The following are recognized features of ulnar nerve lesion of the right elbow:**
    a) Wasting of small muscle of hand.
    b) Loss of sensation of skin of little finger.
    c) Loss of supinator jerk.
    d) Nocturnal pain of the hand.
    e) Abduction of the little finger precedes claw-hand deformity.

46. **Erythema nodosum can be found in the following conditions:**
    a) Systemic lupus erythematosus.
    b) Sarcoidosis.
    c) Herpes simplex infection.
    d) Primary tuberculosis.
    e) Delayed allergic response to beta-haemolytic streptococcal throat infection.

47. **Schizophrenia:**
    a) Is usually seen in the early thirties.
    b) Rarely shows family history of the illness.
    c) Constitutes the majority of long-term mental hospital patients.
    d) May be associated with the feeling of panic while shopping.
    e) Recovery is better if the onset is acute.

48. **The following disorders in time may give rise to malignant changes:**
    a) Chronic duodenal ulcer.
    b) Ulcerative colitis.
    c) Papilloma of the bladder.
    d) Diverticulitis.
    e) Solar keratosis.

49. During the antenatal period:
a) Hypertension, albuminuria and oedema at 14 weeks would be diagnosed as pre-eclampsic toxaemia.
b) All patients should have a chest X-ray to exclude tuberculosis.
c) Cervical cytology is associated with a greater number of false positives.
d) Vaginal examination and assessment should be carried out at 36 weeks.
e) The head should be engaged by 39 weeks in the parous patient.

50. The following are side-effects of the drugs named:
a) Maculopapular rash in more than a third of patients with ampicillin.
b) Aplastic anaemia with chloramphenicol.
c) Eighth cranial nerve damage with streptomycin.
d) Exacerbation of renal failure with tetracycline.
e) Jaundice with erythromycin.

51. The extensor plantar response is a recognized feature in the following:
a) Tabes dorsalis.
b) Subacute combined degeneration of the cord.
c) Hysteria.
d) Syringomyelia.
e) Poliomyelitis.

52. An increase in antidiuretic hormone:
a) Results in decreased serum sodium.
b) Results in decreased creatinine clearance.
c) Can cause epilepsy.
d) Can be found in bronchogenic carcinoma.
e) Is usually treated by fluid restriction.

53. Porphyria cutanea tarda:
a) Is associated with acute abdominal pain.
b) Can be prevented by alcohol.
c) Bullae formation on the skin is a feature.
d) The contraceptive pill is contra-indicated.
e) Venesection is an effective form of treatment.

54. Malignant changes can occur in the following lesions:
   a) Blue naevus.
   b) Pigmented mole.
   c) Adenoma sebaceum.
   d) Albinism.
   e) Xeroderma pigmentosum.

55. Mycosis fungoidus:
   a) Is characteristically commoner in females.
   b) Typically causes atrophy of the skin with reticular pigmentation and telangiectasia.
   c) Is frequently accompanied by splenomegaly.
   d) Causes death within 5 years of diagnosis.
   e) Is caused by a zoophilic fungal infection.

56. The following conditions should arouse suspicion of an underlying malignancy:
   a) Acanthosis nigricans.
   b) Pemphigus vulgaris.
   c) Dermatomyositis.
   d) Alopecia areata.
   e) Persistent figurate erythema.

57. Acanthosis nigricans:
   a) Occurs usually in the axillae and groin.
   b) May be accompanied by warty lesion.
   c) Is usually associated with lymphoma.
   d) The skin changes persist in spite of successful treatment of the internal malignancy.
   e) May occur on the palms and soles.

58. The following features should suggest the possibility of underlying diabetes mellitus:
   a) Balanitis.
   b) Granuloma annulare.
   c) Pyoderma gangrenosum.
   d) Necrobiosis lipoidica.
   e) Bazin's disease.

59. Haematometra is a recognized complication of the following conditions:
a) Failure of Wolffian duct canalization.
b) Persistence of cloacal membrane.
c) Imperforate hymen.
d) Carcinoma of the cervix.
e) Cone biopsy.

60. Regarding oat cell carcinoma of the bronchus:
a) Adrenocorticotrophic hormone secretion can occur.
b) Is commonest cause of pulmonary osteoarthropathy.
c) Antidiuretic hormone secretion may occur.
d) Is a squamous cell carcinoma.
e) Is a small cell carcinoma.

Paper 12   Questions

1. In hepatitis A:
   a) The incubation period is 3–6 months.
   b) The spread is usually by the faeco-oral route.
   c) Jaundice occurs in the majority of patients.
   d) The patient should be advised against drinking alcohol for at least 6 months after the attack.
   e) Oral corticosteroids are the treatment of choice in all cases.

2. In the injured eye:
   a) Pupillary dilatation may occur as the result of a blow to the eye.
   b) Fluorescein colours any corneal abrasion bright orange.
   c) Visual acuity should be assessed at an early stage.
   d) Chemical burns from acids are in general more dangerous than alkalis.
   e) Any possibility of retained foreign body demands urgent ophthalmic opinion.

3. Vitiligo:
   a) Is a fungal infection.
   b) Is associated with alopecia areata.
   c) Does not affect negroes.
   d) Does not resolve spontaneously.
   e) Is best treated by ultraviolet light.

4. Uncomplicated salmonella food poisoning:
   a) Generally comes from food of vegetable origin.
   b) Is caused by organisms which can survive deep-freezing.
   c) Typically presents with vomiting and bloody diarrhoea.
   d) Should be treated with antimicrobial drugs.
   e) Leaves 10% patients as chronic carriers.

5. Lesions of lichen planus:
a) Are characteristically purplish shiny papules.
b) Rarely itch.
c) May occur only in the mouth.
d) On average persist for 6 months.
e) Are usually aggravated by topical application of flourinated steroids.

6. In acute iritis:
a) The pupils are usually constricted.
b) Vision is typically unimpaired.
c) Pain ceases if the eye remains still.
d) Topical steroids are indicated.
e) Mydriatics may help.

7. Ascites is a feature of:
a) Acute pericarditis.
b) Tuberculous peritonitis.
c) Meig's syndrome.
d) Metastatic carcinoma.
e) Alcoholic liver disease.

8. In the treatment of burns it is correct to say:
a) Application of cold water to burned areas relieves pain.
b) Burns from scalds will require more grafting than burns from flames.
c) Children with 10% or more of body surface involvement in burns need hospitalization.
d) Occlusive pressure dressing helps relieve pain.
e) Narcotic analgesics should be avoided.

9. The anterior lobe of the pituitary secretes:
a) Thyroid-stimulating hormone.
b) Growth hormone.
c) Adrenocorticotrophic hormone.
d) Antidiuretic hormone.
e) Thyroid-releasing hormone.

10. Recognized features of neurofibromatosis may include:
   a) Optic atrophy.
   b) Paroxysmal hypertension.
   c) Albuminuria.
   d) Deafness.
   e) Osteosclerosis tibiae.

11. Hypokalaemia is known to occur in:
   a) Excessive purgation.
   b) Cushing's syndrome.
   c) Oliguric renal failure.
   d) Acute hepatitis.
   e) Alkalosis.

12. The following are features of acquired haemolytic anaemia:
   a) Raised conjugated serum bilirubin.
   b) Raised urinary urobilinogen.
   c) Positive Coomb's test.
   d) Raised urinary bilirubin.
   e) Reticulocutosis.

13. In epilepsy the following mental changes may occur:
   a) *Déjà vu* phenomena.
   b) Confused state.
   c) Paranoid delusions.
   d) Mood changes.
   e) Visual hallucinations.

14. Leucopenia is a recognized feature of the following:
   a) Typhoid.
   b) Empyema thoracis.
   c) Systemic lupus erythematosus.
   d) Chloramphenicol therapy.
   e) Haemorrhage.

15. The following are recognized blood changes due to drugs:
   a) Decreased coagulability with aspirin.
   b) Polycythaemia with methyl dopa.
   c) Aplastic anaemia with chloramphenicol.
   d) Haemolytic anaemia with digoxin.
   e) Methaemoglobulinaemia with phenacetin.

16. The following drugs should be used in reduced dosage in chronic renal failure:
   a) Digoxin.
   b) Potassium chloride.
   c) Frusemide.
   d) Intravenous glucose.
   e) Streptomycin.

17. Changes in the sacro-iliac joint may occur in:
   a) Gout.
   b) Ulcerative colitis.
   c) Reiter's disease.
   d) Scleroderma.
   e) Ankylosing spondylitis.

18. Recognized complications of measles include:
   a) Encephalitis.
   b) Otitis media.
   c) Arthritis.
   d) Pneumonia.
   e) Myocarditis.

19. In senile dementia:
   a) The onset is sudden.
   b) Social behaviour is unaffected.
   c) Vasodilators significantly improve memory.
   d) Loss of bowel and bladder control are unusual features.
   e) Mortality is not increased.

20. In the drug treatment of rheumatoid arthritis it is correct to say that:
   a) Tinnitus in patients taking aspirin is a sign for the drug to be stopped at once.
   b) Indomethacin suppositories at night are a useful means of relieving morning stiffness.
   c) Patients receiving gold injections should have regular examinations of their urine.
   d) Soluble aspirin has anti-inflammatory properties at all dosages.
   e) Penicillamine cannot be used in patients who are allergic to penicillin.

21. In normal pregnancy:
   a) The blood urea level rises.
   b) Rising pituitary oxytocin levels are responsible for the initiation of uterine contraction.
   c) Fasting blood sugar levels are greater than in the non-pregnant woman.
   d) Cervical cytology is associated with high false positives.
   e) 300 mcg/d of folic acid is an adequate supplement.

22. Tricyclic antidepressants:
   a) May cause diarrhoea.
   b) Are best combined with barbiturates for the sleepless patient.
   c) Have little placebo effect as compared with drugs used to treat physical condition.
   d) Are useful in phobic states resistant to other treatment.
   e) To be effective should be given three to four times daily at regular intervals.

23. Carcinoma of the ovary:
   a) Is always unilateral.
   b) In the majority of cases presents with abdominal swelling.
   c) Has an overall 5-year survival rate of 60%.
   d) Can now be screened by alpha-fetoprotein studies.
   e) Should nearly always be treated by total hysterectomy with bilateral salpingo-oophorectomy.

24. With a vesico-vaginal fistula:
a) There is increased incidence of urinary tract infection.
b) Continuous wetting is a distressing feature.
c) Faecal incontinence is usually associated.
d) Distended bladder is typically found.
e) Carcinoma of the cervix is a recognized cause.

25. In acute osteomyelitis:
a) Constitutional disturbances are usually seen.
b) Sun-ray specules are characteristically seen in the radiograph.
c) Antibiotics should be started immediately while awaiting blood culture reports.
d) Pus should be drained surgically.
e) Infection can spread to other organs by septic emboli.

26. Characteristic radiological findings in small bowel obstruction are:
a) Air shadow distal to the obstruction.
b) Volvulae conniventes can be clearly seen.
c) Haustration is a radiological hallmark.
d) Distended loops are oriented mainly in the central part of the abdomen.
e) Fluid levels in a supine radiograph are diagnostic.

27. Recognized features of regional ileitis include:
a) Malignancy in long-standing cases.
b) Perianal fistula.
c) Iron deficiency anaemia.
d) Intestinal obstruction.
e) Anal tags and fissures.

28. Hydrocephalus has a known association to:
a) Arnold–Chiari malformation.
b) Aqueduct stenosis.
c) Tuberculous meningitis.
d) Posterior fossa tumour.
e) Subarachnoid haemorrhage.

29. Following are recognized causes of carpal tunnel syndrome:
a) Cervical rib.
b) Acromegaly.
c) Pregnancy.
d) Pneumatic drill worker.
e) Rheumatoid arthritis.

30. Partial gastrectomy was performed in a patient aged 55 years about 10 years ago who is now complaining of backache. Biochemical investigations reveal a low serum calcium and elevated alkaline phophatase. The most likely diagnosis is:
a) Hypoparathyroidism.
b) Hyperparathyroidism.
c) Zollinger–Ellison syndrome.
d) Osteomalacia.
e) Osteoporosis.

31. Hazards associated with spinal anaesthesia can be seen in:
a) Torsion of the testis.
b) Psoriasis.
c) Sickle cell anaemia.
d) Porphyria.
e) Acute alcohol intoxication.

32. A 60-year-old woman has acute severe haematemesis. There is no past history of bleeding or indigestion. Management should include:
a) Measurement of plasma factor eight level.
b) Measurement of plasma albumin level.
c) Examination of stools for occult blood.
d) Emergency opaque meal radiological examination if gastroduodenoscopy is not available.
e) Emergency gastroduodenography if available.

33. Recognized causes of earache include:
a) Otosclerosis.
b) Carcinoma of the pharynx.
c) Otitis externa.
d) Perichondritis of the pinna.
e) Dental caries.

34. The signs of severe shock include:
a) Pallor.
b) Elevated blood pressure.
c) Increased pulse rate.
d) Cold moist skin.
e) Increased excretion of urine.

35. Features of Cushing's syndrome include:
a) Obesity.
b) Hypertension.
c) Hypogonadism.
d) Glycosuria.
e) Diarrhoea.

36. Vitamin K:
a) Is required for normal prothrombin formation.
b) Is used pre-operatively in obstructive jaundice.
c) Deficiency causes a positive capillary fragility test.
d) Is useful in treatment of haemophilia.
e) May cause metastatic calcification.

37. In a new-born:
a) The ductus arteriosus closes immediately after delivery.
b) The bowel is sterile.
c) Pulse rate of 70–80 per minute.
d) There is physiological jaundice between 6–8 days.
e) Nasolacrimal duct is open at birth.

38. Progressive dysphagia is seen in:
    a) Bulbar palsy.
    b) Carcinoma of the hypopharynx.
    c) Muscular dystrophy.
    d) Myasthenia gravis.
    e) Peritonsillar abscess.

39. The following are recognized features of the Paterson–Kelly syndrome:
    a) Koilonychia.
    b) Increased haemoglobin concentration.
    c) Hyperchlorhydria.
    d) Elderly men are commonly affected.
    e) Achlorhydria.

40. Intraepithelial carcinoma of the cervix:
    a) Is usually associated with positive cytology.
    b) Does not cross the basement membrane.
    c) Histology shows carcinomatous cells.
    d) Extends to cervical glands.
    e) First line of treatment is cone biopsy.

41. Causes of hypokalaemia include:
    a) Spironolactone therapy.
    b) Thiazide treatment.
    c) Conn's syndrome.
    d) Addison's disease.
    e) Gastrointestinal fistula.

42. Plasma volume is found to be severely depleted in:
    a) Burns.
    b) Pyloric stenosis.
    c) Slow blood loss.
    d) Frusemide therapy.
    e) Huge strangulated hernia.

43. Recognized causes of raised alkaline phosphatase include:
a) Osteitis fibrosa cystica.
b) Renal osteodystrophy.
c) Osteomalacia.
d) Osteoarthritis.
e) Amyloidosis.

44. In retrobulbar neuritis:
a) There may be pain in the eye.
b) Tunnel vision is a recognized consequence.
c) The blind spot may be enlarged.
d) Smoking is a known cause.
e) Multiple sclerosis may be the cause.

45. Causes of sustained diastolic hypertension in a young woman include:
a) Femoral artery stenosis.
b) Coarctation of aorta.
c) Patent ductus arteriosus.
d) Phaeochromocytoma.
e) Thyrotoxicosis.

46. Carcinoma of the large bowel:
a) Is more common in the right than in the left colon.
b) Is the commonest cause of acute large bowel obstruction.
c) Is a common cause of iron deficiency anaemia.
d) Is a recognized complication of chronic ulcerative colitis.
e) Always requires the establishment of colonoscopy.

47. Recognized causes of melaena include:
a) Rectal cancer.
b) Crohn's disease.
c) Aspirin ingestion.
d) Hiatus hernia.
e) Oral iron treatment.

48. The following are known causes of pulsatile fistula:
   a) Thyrotoxicosis.
   b) Carotico-cavernous fistula.
   c) Paget's disease of the bone.
   d) Internal carotid artery occlusion.
   e) Aneurysm of posterior communicating artery.

49. Complications of regional ileitis include:
   a) Enteroenteric fistula formation.
   b) Recurrence following excision of the primary lesion.
   c) Fistula in ano.
   d) Malignant change.
   e) Perforation.

50. Secondary amenorrhoea is associated with:
   a) Anorexia nervosa.
   b) Menopause.
   c) Leiomyoma.
   d) Thyrotoxicosis.
   e) Endometriosis.

51. Conditions that may give rise to locking of the knee include:
   a) Torn medial meniscus.
   b) Recurrent dislocation of the patella.
   c) Tibial tubercle apophysitis.
   d) Torn anterior cruciate ligament.
   e) Loose bodies in the joint.

52. Trichomonas vaginitis:
   a) Is a sexually transmitted disease.
   b) Responds to metronidazole.
   c) Predisposes to vulval carcinoma.
   d) Predisposes to Bartholin's abscess.
   e) Can be diagnosed by exfoliative cytology.

53. The following are associated with a raised incidence of pre-eclampsic toxaemia:
a) Maternal smoking in pregnancy.
b) Multiparity.
c) Twin pregnancy.
d) Consanguineous marriage.
e) Hydatidiform mole.

54. Cervical erosion:
a) Commonly occurs during pregnancy.
b) May be diagnosed by cervical cytology.
c) Is a cause of intermenstrual bleeding.
d) Is usually covered by squamous epithelium.
e) May be treated by cryosurgery.

55. Forceps delivery is indicated in:
a) Cord prolapse with cervix fully dilated.
b) Occipito-posterior position at the onset of second stage.
c) Failure to progress in the second stage with the head not yet engaged.
d) Premature delivery at 32 weeks.
e) Cases of epidural anaesthesia.

56. A non-pregnant 40-year-old woman has a 10 cm diameter swelling discovered on routine examination of the pelvis:
a) It is probably hydrosalpinx.
b) The patient should be examined in 3 months' time.
c) Exploratory laparotomy may be required.
d) A colposcopy should be performed.
e) The exact cause is investigated by examination under anaesthesia.

57. Unstable lie in late pregnancy:
a) May be caused by bicornuate uterus.
b) Is not hazardous if associated with high parity.
c) May be associated with fetal abnormality.
d) Is an indication for hospital admission before term.
e) May be associated with placenta praevia.

58. Adenomyosis:
   a) Is a condition where endometrial tissue is found within the myometrium.
   b) Frequently presents with dysmenorrhoea.
   c) Is often associated with amenorrhoea.
   d) May occur within a uterine fibroid.
   e) Usually predisposes to myometrial leiomyosarcoma.

59. Endometrial carcinoma:
   a) Is a cause of postmenopausal bleeding.
   b) Occurs in an older age group than carcinoma of the cervix.
   c) Is usually a squamous cell carcinoma.
   d) Is more common than carcinoma of the cervix.
   e) Is the single most common malignancy in women.

60. Precipitate labour is associated with:
   a) Increased infant mortality rate.
   b) Cervical incompetence.
   c) Perineal tear.
   d) Maternal pulmonary tuberculosis.
   e) Post-partum haemorrhage.

Paper 13   Questions

1. Left ventricular failure is a recognized feature of the following:
   a) Systemic hypertension.
   b) Mitral stenosis.
   c) Coarctation of aorta.
   d) Aortic incompetence.
   e) Atrial septal defect.

2. Cholestatic jaundice may complicate therapy with:
   a) Streptomycin.
   b) Chlorpromazine.
   c) Warfarin.
   d) Methyl testosterone.
   e) Phenobarbitone.

3. Human immunoglobulins are useful in the following:
   a) Measles.
   b) Infectious hepatitis.
   c) Rhesus immunization.
   d) Tuberculosis.
   e) Rubella.

4. The following drugs can be used to avoid premature labour:
   a) Ethanol.
   b) Indomethacin.
   c) Propranolol.
   d) Hydrallazine.
   e) Salbutamol.

5. **Recognized features of multiple sclerosis include:**
   a) Double vision.
   b) Telangiectasia of face.
   c) Difficulty in micturition.
   d) Difficulty in swallowing.
   e) Sore throat.

6. **Hypercapnia is a characteristic feature of the following:**
   a) Chronic bronchitis.
   b) Diabetic ketoacidosis.
   c) Acute bronchial asthma.
   d) Severe barbiturate poisoning.
   e) Hysteria.

7. **Complications associated with pyloric obstruction may include:**
   a) Acidosis.
   b) Diarrhoea.
   c) Hyperkalaemia.
   d) Oliguria.
   e) Hypochloraemia.

8. **The following features may be found in uncomplicated patent ductus arteriosus:**
   a) Left to right shunt.
   b) Increased pulmonary artery pressure.
   c) Machinery-like murmur.
   d) Cyanosis.
   e) Cardiac enlargement.

9. **The following have a recognized association with giant cell arteritis:**
   a) Sudden loss of visual acuity.
   b) Very high erythrocyte sedimentation rate.
   c) Hemicranial pain.
   d) Cataract of rapid onset.
   e) Subconjunctival haemorrhage.

10. Megaloblastic anaemia may complicate the following therapy:
a) Phenobarbitone.
b) Phenytoin sodium.
c) Phenindione.
d) Paracetamol.
e) Primidone.

11. Increased alkaline phosphatase is characteristically found in the following conditions:
a) Osteomalacia.
b) Myocardial infarction.
c) Osteitis fibrosa cystica.
d) Azotemic renal dystrophy.
e) Ankylosing spondylitis.

12. Deafness is a recognized complication of the following therapy:
a) Streptomycin.
b) Frusemide.
c) Aspirin.
d) Tetracycline.
e) Quinine.

13. Features of occlusion of the right middle cerebral artery in a right-handed person can include:
a) Left homonymous hemianopia.
b) Expressive dysphasia.
c) Paraplegia.
d) Right horizontal nystagmus.
e) Bitemporal hemianopia.

14. The following are true of untreated Parkinsonism:
a) Intension tremor.
b) Cog-wheel rigidity.
c) Absent ankle jerk.
d) Infrequent blinking.
e) Positive Rhomberg's sign.

15. Appropriate treatment of post-partum haemorrhage includes:
a) Vaginal packing.
b) Uterine packing.
c) Uterine exploration.
d) Intravenous ergotamine.
e) Laparotomy.

16. The following physical signs are correctly associated with fat embolism:
a) Delirium.
b) Hypothermia.
c) Petechiae.
d) Dyspnoea.
e) Xanthomata.

17. In a supracondylar fracture in a child:
a) Arm should be immobilized in flexion.
b) Can be immobilized in extension.
c) There may be associated arterial injury.
d) Non-union is a known complication.
e) Median and ulnar nerve involvement are rare complications.

18. The terminal interphalangeal joint is typically involved in the following diseases:
a) Osteoarthritis.
b) Psoriatic arthritis.
c) Rheumatoid arthritis.
d) Tubercular arthritis.
e) Reiter's disease.

19. The first stage of labour can be shortened by:
a) Artificial rupture of membranes.
b) Oxytocin drip.
c) Intravenous ergometrine.
d) Forceps delivery.
e) Caesarean section.

20. Features of aortic stenosis include:
a) Angina.
b) Apical diastolic murmur.
c) Basal systolic murmur.
d) Increased peripheral pulsation.
e) Accentuated second heart sound.

21. Ectopic pregnancy:
a) Is commonest in the ampullary region.
b) Shows a higher chance of recurrence.
c) Can be confused with unilateral pelvic inflammation.
d) Shows secretory endometrium in the uterus.
e) Can be successfully treated with laparoscopy.

22. The following are recognized features of Cushing's syndrome:
a) Hypertension.
b) Psychiatric symptomatology.
c) Retardation of sexual development.
d) Hirsutism.
e) Polycythaemia.

23. Transverse lie may occur in:
a) Placenta praevia.
b) Bicornuate uterus.
c) Arcuate uterus.
d) Twin pregnancy.
e) Mongolism.

24. The following factors enhance the chances of vaginal delivery in a patient who had a previous caesarean section:
a) Elective caesarean section at the previous pregnancy.
b) A non-recurrent cause was the indication for caesarean section.
c) Emergency caesarean section in the previous pregnancy.
d) Normal hysterogram in between previous and present pregnancy.
e) One normal vaginal delivery subsequent to the first caesarean section.

25. **In utero-vaginal prolapse:**
   a) An elongated cervix is often present.
   b) The transverse cervical ligament which supports the vaginal wall is weak.
   c) Overflow incontinence may be seen.
   d) A pessary is useful in the treatment.
   e) Pelvic floor exercises are useful in severe cases.

26. **Biguanides:**
   a) Act by stimulating insulin secretion.
   b) Often cause photosensitivity.
   c) Are usually used in juvenile diabetes mellitus.
   d) Can be used in obesity.
   e) Are known to cause lactic acidosis.

27. **The second stage of carcinoma of the cervix:**
   a) Is usually clinically detectable.
   b) Is an invasive carcinoma.
   c) Is a malignant condition.
   d) Could be diagnosed by cytology.
   e) Basement membrane is typically intact.

28. **Urinary protein excretion of 15 g per day is consistent with:**
   a) Diabetic nephropathy.
   b) Chronic industrial exposure to mercury.
   c) Chronic pyelonephritis.
   d) Adult Fanconi syndrome.
   e) Type 1 renal tubular acidosis.

29. **A raised diaphragm on a chest X-ray is seen in the following conditions:**
   a) Pulmonary infarction.
   b) Chronic bronchitis.
   c) Tuberculosis.
   d) Enlarged liver.
   e) Left ventricular failure.

30. In schizophrenia:
a) Visual hallucinations are common.
b) Thought blocks may occur.
c) Auditory hallucinations may take the form of abusive senseless phrases.
d) Familial incidence is recognized.
e) Phenothiazines may be indicated.

31. Vitamin B$_{12}$ deficiency is a recognized complication of the following conditions:
a) Diphyllobothrium latum infestation.
b) Jejunal diverticulosis.
c) Pregnancy.
d) Phenytoin therapy.
e) Malnutrition.

32. Petit mal epilepsy:
a) Usually begins in early adolescence.
b) Is characterized by tongue biting during the attack.
c) Is commonly associated with migraine.
d) Has a characteristic EEG with a spike and wave form at 30 cycles per second.
e) Attack may be followed by automatism.

33. The following statements are true:
a) The ulnar nerve supplies the majority of the flexor muscles in the forearm.
b) The ulnar nerve supplies the intrinsic muscles of the hand.
c) The median nerve supplies the hypothenar muscles.
d) The radial nerve supplies the dorsal interossei.
e) The radial nerve supplies the majority of the extensor muscles of the forearm.

34. Raised intracranial pressure is suggested by the following:
a) Photophobia.
b) Blurring of vision.
c) Neck stiffness and positive Kernig's sign.
d) Headache characteristically present on walking.
e) Nausea.

35. Recognized features of nutritional rickets include:
   a) Craniotabes.
   b) Subperiosteal haemorrhage.
   c) Raised phosphorus level.
   d) Reduced alkaline phosphatase.
   e) Defective calcification of long bones.

36. The following are true of calculus in the submandibular gland:
   a) Presence of painful swelling for 2–3 weeks.
   b) There may be pain on eating.
   c) May present as a hard mass in the floor of the mouth.
   d) Usually shows characteristic opacity of X-ray.
   e) Sialography typically shows punctate sialectasis.

37. In depression:
   a) Paranoid delusions are common.
   b) Early morning awakening is characteristic.
   c) There may be loss of libido.
   d) Memory for recent events is poor.
   e) Tricyclic antidepressants may show adrenergic side-effects.

38. Carpal tunnel syndrome occurs in the following conditions:
   a) Syringomyelia.
   b) Pregnancy.
   c) Myxoedema.
   d) Rheumatoid arthritis.
   e) Gout.

39. Schizophrenia:
   a) Occurs in 0.5% of the general population.
   b) Eventually always requires hospitalization.
   c) May be familial.
   d) Is frequently associated with social withdrawal and hallucinations.
   e) May be induced by drugs.

40. Causes of sudden blindness include:
a) Vitreous haemorrhage.
b) Choroidoretinitis of toxoplasmosis.
c) Temporal arteritis.
d) Glaucoma.
e) Neurosyphilis.

41. In the following conditions ascites is usually present on clinical examination:
a) Left ventricular failure.
b) Cirrhosis.
c) Intra-abdominal Hodgkin's disease.
d) Nephrotic syndrome.
e) Carcinoma of the uterus.

42. Untoward effects associated with use of beta-blocker therapy include:
a) Congestive cardiac failure.
b) Hyperglycaemia.
c) Arrhythmias.
d) Asthma.
e) Heart block.

43. The following are recognized features of systemic lupus erythematosus:
a) Thrombocytopenia.
b) Fits.
c) Pericardial friction rub.
d) Plate-like atelectasis on chest X-ray.
e) Isolated pleural effusion.

44. Features of premature infants include:
a) Weight less than 2500 g.
b) Susceptibility to birth trauma.
c) Hypoglycaemia.
d) Hypothermia.
e) Dry wrinkled skin.

45. The following commonly occur in left ventricular failure:
a) Paroxysmal nocturnal dyspnoea.
b) Fine bilateral basal crepitations.
c) Right-sided pleural effusion.
d) Reversed splitting of the second sound.
e) Splenomegaly.

46. Pernicious anaemia is associated with:
a) Antibodies to parietal cells.
b) Antibodies to intrinsic factor.
c) Antibodies to thyroid cytoplasm.
d) Antibodies to mitochondria.
e) Antibodies to smooth muscle.

47. The following features are typical of mitral stenosis:
a) Mid-diastolic rumbling murmur.
b) Opening snap just following the first sound.
c) Loud first heart sound.
d) Recurrent chest infection.
e) Relative reduction in blood flow to apices of the lung.

48. Jaundice with pale stools and dark urine is characteristic of the following conditions:
a) Infectious hepatitis.
b) Pancreatic carcinoma.
c) Hepatoma.
d) Glandular fever hepatitis.
e) Primary biliary cirrhosis.

49. The following are likely causes of acute abdominal pain and rectal bleeding in the elderly:
a) Haemorrhoids.
b) Hepatoma.
c) Diverticular disease.
d) Ulcerative colitis.
e) Carcinoma of the colon.

50. Recognized features of tuberculosis of the spine include:
a) Scoliosis.
b) Kyphosis.
c) Lower motor neurone signs.
d) Psoas muscle spasm.
e) Vertebral collapse.

51. The following are useful in the treatment of pulmonary oedema:
a) Posture.
b) Oxygen.
c) Frusemide.
d) Beta-2 stimulant.
e) Heroin.

52. Hypercalcaemia is a recognized complication of the following conditions:
a) Multiple myeloma.
b) Hypoparathyroidism.
c) Senile osteoporosis.
d) Sarcoidosis.
e) Lack of vitamin D.

53. Normocytic normochromic anaemia is known to occur in:
a) Uraemia.
b) Folate deficiency.
c) Secondaries in bone marrow.
d) Hereditary elliptocytosis.
e) Splenectomy.

54. A lung abscess is a recognized complication of the following conditions:
a) Heroin addiction.
b) Acute osteomyelitis.
c) Achalasia cardia.
d) Mycoplasma pneumonia.
e) Staphylococcus pneumonia.

55. **Purpura without reduced platelet count may occur in the following conditions:**
    a) Elderly people.
    b) Acute lymphoblastic leukaemia.
    c) Aplastic anaemia.
    d) Henoch–Schoenlein purpura.
    e) Patients on steroids.

56. **Complications of diabetes mellitus include:**
    a) Nephrotic syndrome.
    b) Pruritus vulvae.
    c) Third nerve palsy.
    d) Sarcoidosis.
    e) Perforating foot ulcer.

57. **Megaloblastic anaemia is a recognized complication of the following conditions:**
    a) Ulcerative colitis.
    b) Amoebic dysentery.
    c) Crohn's disease.
    d) Coeliac disease.
    e) Chronic pancreatitis.

58. **Generalized lymphadenopathy is characteristic of the following conditions:**
    a) Bacillary dysentery.
    b) Schistosomiasis.
    c) Toxoplasmosis.
    d) Tuberculosis.
    e) Recurrent malaria.

59. **The following are characteristic features of hypopituitarism:**
    a) Reduced axillary hair.
    b) Rough skin.
    c) Pigmentation of skin.
    d) Delayed puberty.
    e) Amenorrhoea.

60. Disseminated intravascular coagulation is a recognized complication of the following:
   a) Gram-negative septicaemia.
   b) Polycythaemia rubra vera.
   c) Transplant rejection.
   d) Incompatible blood transfusion.
   e) Oral contraceptive.

Paper 14   Questions

1. Abortion:

a) Generally presents as bleeding followed by pain.
b) Before 12 weeks in the majority of cases is due to chromosomal abnormality.
c) If threatened and followed by pregnancy to term then it is not associated with an increased risk to the fetus.
d) If recurrent before 12–14 weeks implies cervical incompetence.
e) May be followed by choriocarcinoma.

2. Cannon waves in the jugular venous pressure are:

a) A special form of 'v' wave.
b) Seen in complete heart block.
c) Seen in tricuspid stenosis.
d) Compatible with nodal rhythm.
e) Associated with second degree heart block.

3. A marked elevation in the levels of serum gastrin is seen in:

a) Zollinger–Ellison syndrome.
b) Duodenal ulcer.
c) Pernicious anaemia.
d) Gastric ulcer.
e) Pyloric stenosis.

4. Retroperitoneal fibrosis may present as:

a) Chronic renal failure.
b) Biliary colic.
c) Sterility in young women.
d) Leg oedema without raised jugular venous pressure.
e) A result of migraine treatment.

5. In the drug treatment of rheumatoid arthritis:
   a) Paracetamol has only a mild anti-inflammatory effect.
   b) Pain may be temporarily increased if indomethacin is suddenly stopped.
   c) Chloroquine is safe provided the retinae are checked every 3 months.
   d) Gold salts give immediate benefit.
   e) Phenylbutazone should not be given if there is a past history of peptic ulceration.

6. Cheyne–Stokes breathing is a feature of the following conditions:
   a) Uraemia.
   b) Head injury.
   c) Meningitis.
   d) Diabetic coma.
   e) Hypoxic encephalopathy.

7. Polyhydramnios is a recognized complication of the following:
   a) Meningocele.
   b) Diabetic mother.
   c) Imperforate anus.
   d) Oesophageal atresia.
   e) Post-maturity.

8. Recognized features of acromegaly include:
   a) Bitemporal hemianopia.
   b) Thickening of the heel pad and tufting of the terminal phalanges.
   c) Raised levels of growth hormone which can be suppressed with glucose.
   d) Hypertension in 40% of patients.
   e) Excessive perspiration.

9. **The following complications can occur in rheumatoid arthritis:**
   a) Acanthosis nigricans.
   b) Episcleritis.
   c) Malabsorption.
   d) Carpal tunnel syndrome.
   e) Amyloidosis.

10. **Anaemia in pregnancy:**
   a) May result in heart failure.
   b) May cause fetal hypoxia as a complication.
   c) Can occur due to threadworm infestation.
   d) May be treated effectively with parenteral iron.
   e) Is a recognized complication of malaria.

11. **The following complications definitely improve with control of diabetes mellitus:**
   a) Peripheral neuropathy.
   b) Mononeuritis multiplex.
   c) Vulvo-vaginitis.
   d) Proximal amyotrophy.
   e) Angina.

12. **In Cushing's syndrome:**
   a) Adrenal adenoma is present in 20% of cases.
   b) Adrenal adenoma is present in 10% of cases.
   c) Hyperpigmentation is present in buccal mucosa.
   d) Confusion may occur.
   e) Proximal myopathy can occur.

13. **The following complicate steroid therapy:**
   a) Vitiligo.
   b) Diabetes mellitus.
   c) Anhydrosis.
   d) Osteoporosis.
   e) Hypercalcaemia.

14. Ptosis of the eyelids is a feature of:
   a) Myasthenia gravis.
   b) Tabes dorsalis.
   c) Fifth cranial nerve palsy.
   d) Trigeminal neuralgia.
   e) Third cranial nerve palsy.

15. Deterioration in a patient with head injury is determined by:
   a) Serial EEGs.
   b) Deepening conscious level.
   c) Repeated angiography.
   d) Pupils becoming fixed.
   e) Computerized axial tomography.

16. Recognized features of acute appendicitis include:
   a) Feter oris.
   b) Diarrhoea.
   c) Shifting of pain from umbilicus to right iliac fossa.
   d) Leucoplakia.
   e) Furred tongue.

17. A woman of 56 years presents with haematuria. Which of the following would be likely causes?:
   a) Bleeding disorder.
   b) Urinary infection.
   c) Cystinuria.
   d) Bladder tumour.
   e) Cushing's syndrome.

18. The following clinical features are common in patients in shock:
   a) Peripheral cyanosis.
   b) Sweating.
   c) Purpura.
   d) Thirst.
   e) Cheyne–Stokes breathing.

19. Acute prostatitis:
   a) Commonly leads to rigors.
   b) May be due to Neisserian gonorrhoea.
   c) Usually presents as perineal pain and dysuria.
   d) Typically requires drainage with a resectoscope.
   e) Rectal examination commonly reveals a hard craggy mass.

20. The following are recognized features of severe accidental haemorrhage:
   a) Free presenting part.
   b) Painful vaginal bleeding.
   c) Tender uterus.
   d) Absent fetal heart sound.
   e) Maternal shock.

21. In a Colles' fracture displacement of the distal fragment includes:
   a) Rotation posteriorly.
   b) Ulnar deviation.
   c) Supination.
   d) Impaction to the radial side.
   e) Pronation.

22. A diameter of more than 9.5 cm at term is found in the following position:
   a) Suboccipito bregmatic.
   b) Occipito frontal.
   c) Submento bregmatic.
   d) Biparietal diameter.
   e) Submento vertical.

23. A depressed patient may show:
   a) Agitation.
   b) Decreased ability to concentrate.
   c) Hallucination.
   d) Weight loss.
   e) Decreased facial expression.

24. Dupuytren's contracture:
a) Is due to contracted flexor tendons.
b) Is due to contraction of the palmar fascia.
c) Seldom affects the ring finger.
d) Is commoner in males.
e) Is usually cured with stretching and splinting.

25. In a 50-year-old man with a blood pressure of 180/115 on three separate recordings:
a) Right ventricular hypertrophy may be present.
b) Arterio-venous nipping would suggest that the hypertension is not of recent onset.
c) Intravenous pyelography would be an appropriate first line of investigation.
d) The aim of the treatment is to get his blood pressure to 120/80 immediately.
e) Guanethidine as an anti-hypertensive may lead to failure of ejaculation.

26. Psoriasis:
a) Is caused in half of acute cases by a delayed allergic reaction to beta-haemolyic streptococcal throat infection.
b) Affects nearly 2% of the general population of the UK.
c) Rarely involves the nails.
d) Is often greatly helped by a course of ultraviolet light in a suberythemal dosage.
e) Is one condition where oral steroids have virtually no role in the management.

27. Post-operative deep vein thrombosis:
a) Does not occur until 7 days after operation.
b) Is presently undetected clinically.
c) When arising in the solar plexus is most likely to lead to pulmonary embolism.
d) Is often accompanied by superficial thrombophlebitis.
e) May be prevented by heparin prophylaxis.

28. Recognized features of a strangulated hernia include:
a) Tense on palpation.
b) Tender on palpation.
c) Is resonant on percussion.
d) Has no expansile impulse on coughing.
e) Is transilluminant.

29. A patient who ingested 20 g of paracetamol:
a) May look and feel well initially.
b) Is likely to develop indigestion.
c) Should have plasma paracetamol levels monitored.
d) May be treated at home after administration of emetics.
e) May develop severe hepatic failure without developing jaundice.

30. Features associated with an arterio-venous fistula include:
a) Increased pulse pressure.
b) Increased cardiac output.
c) Can cause distal gangrene.
d) Reduced central venous pressure.
e) Growth retardation of the limb.

31. Distension of the gall bladder occurs in association with carcinoma of the :
a) Ampulla of Vater.
b) Hepatic ducts.
c) Common bile ducts.
d) Duodenum.
e) Head of the pancreas.

32. Carcinoma of the large bowel:
a) Is commoner in the right than in the left.
b) Is the commonest cause of acute large bowel obstruction.
c) Is a common cause of iron deficiency anaemia.
d) Is a recognized complication of chronic ulcerative colitis.
e) Always requires colostomy.

33. Results of investigations of a patient with 36 h of vomiting due to pyloric stenosis include:
   a) Increased haematocrit.
   b) Increased plasma bicarbonate concentration.
   c) Reduced plasma pH.
   d) Neutral gastric aspirate.
   e) Increased plasma chloride concentration.

34. Haemochromatosis:
   a) Is common in women.
   b) Causes loss of body hair.
   c) May cause heart failure.
   d) May cause hyperuricaemic gout.
   e) Can be treated with reduced iron intake.

35. Increased incidence of carcinoma of the stomach is found in the following conditions:
   a) Pernicious anaemia.
   b) O blood group.
   c) Crohn's disease.
   d) Duodenal ulcer.
   e) Achlorhydria.

36. Liver abscesses can occur in the following:
   a) Amoebic dysentery.
   b) Leptospirosis.
   c) Hepatitis.
   d) Acute appendicitis.
   e) Brucellosis.

37. Recognized features of cystic fibrosis include:
   a) Steatorrhoea.
   b) Hypokalaemia.
   c) Increased sweat sodium.
   d) Chronic productive cough.
   e) Jaundice.

38. **The following are recognized features of rheumatic fever:**
    a) First degree heart block.
    b) Pericarditis.
    c) Painless subcutaneous nodules.
    d) Erythema multiforme.
    e) Erythema marginatum.

39. **An embolus completely obstructing the pulmonary artery:**
    a) Usually occurs in 30% of patients after pelvic surgery.
    b) May cause reduced pressure in left atria.
    c) Can cause pulmonary hypertension.
    d) Typically causes collapse of lobe it supplies.
    e) Causes complete necrosis in the area.

40. **Acute extracellular fluid depletion causes:**
    a) Increased blood urea.
    b) Increased urine osmolality.
    c) Reduced skin elasticity.
    d) Raised haematocrit.
    e) Raised specific gravity of urine.

41. **The following are recognized features of right middle cerebral artery occlusion in a right-handed person:**
    a) Expressive dysphasia.
    b) Left homonymous hemianopia.
    c) Loss of proprioception.
    d) Paraplegia.
    e) Horner's syndrome.

42. **Karyotyping is useful in the diagnosis of the following conditions:**
    a) Sickle cell disease.
    b) Turner's syndrome.
    c) Klinefelter's syndrome.
    d) Cystic fibrosis.
    e) Thalassaemia.

43. Manifestations of hypovolaemia include:
a) Low central venous pressure.
b) Raised catecholamines.
c) Reduced skin elasticity.
d) Raised haematocrit.
e) Raised specific gravity of urine.

44. Cerebrospinal fluid is normal in the following conditions:
a) Syringomyelia.
b) Spinal tumour.
c) Parkinson's disease.
d) Acoustic nerve tumour.
e) Guillain–Barré syndrome.

45. Characteristic features of pain in acute salpingitis include:
a) Colicky.
b) Central.
c) Radiates to umbilicus.
d) Worse on intercourse.
e) Associated with headache.

46. The diagnosis of secondary infertility indicates that:
a) Sterility is secondary to a medical condition.
b) No living children have been produced.
c) Pregnancy has previously occurred.
d) The infertility is reversible.
e) The infertility can be due to secondary syphilis.

47. Contra-indications to oral contraceptives include:
a) Varicose veins.
b) Generalized pruritus in a previous pregnancy.
c) Carcinoma of the breast.
d) Menorrhagia.
e) Previous history of thromboembolism.

48. **The following conditions are contra-indications for external cephalic version:**
    a) Scar in the uterus.
    b) Rhesus incompatibility.
    c) Hypertension.
    d) After 36 weeks.
    e) Anaesthesia.

49. **Post-partum shock without excessive blood loss may occur in the following:**
    a) Acute inversion of the uterus.
    b) Accidental intravenous ergometrine.
    c) Rupture of the uterus.
    d) Paravaginal haematoma.
    e) Third degree tear.

50. **The following are true of first trimester bleeding:**
    a) In threatened abortion pain precedes bleeding.
    b) Vaginal bleeding and uterine size large for date are found in hydatidiform mole.
    c) Shoulder pain may indicate ectopic pregnancy.
    d) Ectopic pregnancy is indicated by profuse bleeding.
    e) Ectopic pregnancy can be confirmed under general anaesthesia.

51. **Secreting ovarian tumours produce:**
    a) Vasopressin.
    b) Thyroxine.
    c) Oestrogen.
    d) Androgen.
    e) Gonadotrophins.

52. **Recognized causes of vulval irritation include:**
    a) Carcinoma of the body of the uterus.
    b) Acute bartholinitis.
    c) Trichomonas vaginitis.
    d) Cervical erosion.
    e) Excessive clothing.

53. Carcinoma of the bronchus may present as:
a) Cushing's syndrome.
b) Peripheral neuropathy.
c) Epilepsy.
d) Cor pulmonale.
e) Amyloidosis.

54. Cyanosis is a recognized feature of the following conditions:
a) Fallot's tetralogy.
b) Pulmonary stenosis.
c) Atrial septal defect.
d) Ventricular septal defect.
e) Patent ductus uterus.

55. Features of a prolapsed disc involving the L3 root include:
a) Pain on coughing.
b) Depressed ankle jerk.
c) Foot drop.
d) Diminished sensitivity of dorsum of foot.
e) Limitation of leg raising.

56. Manifestations of thyrotoxicosis include:
a) Proximal myopathy.
b) Atrial fibrillation.
c) Ophthalmoplegia.
d) Peripheral neuropathy.
e) Tremors.

57. In laceration of soft tissue of the leg routine management includes:
a) Administration of antitetanus serum.
b) Systemic antibiotic.
c) Primary closure.
d) Radiography of the limb.
e) Debridement of wound.

58. A white cell count of more than 17 000 per mm^3 and jaundice are recognized in the following conditions:
   a) Leptospirosis.
   b) Hepatitis.
   c) Primary or secondary tumours of the liver.
   d) Suppurative conjunctivitis.
   e) Appendicitis.

59. Typical features of motor neurone disease include:
   a) Muscle wasting.
   b) Fasciculations.
   c) Optic neuritis.
   d) Papilloedema.
   e) Dissociated anaesthesia.

60. Abruptio placenta is associated with the following features:
   a) Albuminuria.
   b) Absence of pain.
   c) Tenderness over body of uterus.
   d) Fetal malpresentation.
   e) Features of shock out of proportion to blood loss.

Paper 15   Questions

1. In silicosis:
   a) Clubbing can occur.
   b) Can be complicated by tuberculosis.
   c) Progressive fibrosis is a recognized complication.
   d) X-ray findings may resemble tuberculosis.
   e) Mesothelioma can occur.

2. Recognized features of tabes dorsalis include:
   a) Dilated pupil.
   b) Ptosis.
   c) Decreased reflexes.
   d) Loss of sensation.
   e) Charcot's joints.

3. Post-coital bleeding is a known manifestation of the following:
   a) Erosion of the cervix.
   b) Carcinoma of the cervix.
   c) Endometriosis.
   d) Cervical polyp.
   e) Pelvic inflammatory disease.

4. A patient with hypoproteinaemia and cirrhosis develops aberrant behaviour. Appropriate treatment includes:
   a) Neomycin.
   b) Phenytoin.
   c) Reduced protein intake.
   d) MAOI.
   e) Fresh plasma infusion.

5. **Chronic pancreatitis is a recognized manifestation of the following conditions:**
   a) Hyperlipidaemia.
   b) Hyperparathyroidism.
   c) Chronic alcohol abuse.
   d) Insulin-dependent diabetes mellitus.
   e) Gallstones.

6. **Collapsing pulse is a sign seen in:**
   a) Mitral stenosis.
   b) Thyrotoxicosis.
   c) Arterio-venous malformation.
   d) Aortic incompetence.
   e) Patent ductus arteriosus.

7. **In porphyria:**
   a) Abnormal mentation can occur.
   b) Barbiturates are useful.
   c) Photosensitivity of the skin is a recognized manifestation.
   d) Haematuria typically occurs.
   e) Clinical features may mimic lead poisoning.

8. **Bladder tumour:**
   a) Is rarely malignant.
   b) May result from exposure to aniline dye.
   c) May present as painless haematuria.
   d) Can be caused by bilharziasis.
   e) Can arise from a precancerous condition like leukoplakia.

9. **Left ventricular hypertrophy is known to occur in:**
   a) Mitral stenosis.
   b) Aortic incompetence.
   c) Tricuspid stenosis.
   d) Atrial stenosis.
   e) Mitral incompetence.

10. Recognized features of hypothermia include:
a) Acidosis.
b) Hypotension.
c) Ventricular fibrillation.
d) Acute pancreatitis.
e) Hypoglycaemia.

11. A trachea deviated to the right may be seen in:
a) Left pleural effusion.
b) Right pneumothorax.
c) Right upper bronchus obstruction.
d) Left consolidation.
e) Left fibrosis.

12. Excessive loss of plasma may be associated with the following:
a) Slow bleeding.
b) Burns.
c) Strangulated hernia.
d) Surgical wound.
e) Surgical shock.

13. Causes of bulging anterior fontanelle include:
a) Cretinism.
b) Raised intracranial tension.
c) Hydrocephalus.
d) Meningitis.
e) Rickets.

14. Eighth nerve damage may occur with the following therapy:
a) Kanamycin.
b) Erythromycin.
c) Gentamycin.
d) Streptomycin.
e) Tobramycin.

15. Factors predisposing to acute renal failure include:
a) Severe hypoperfusion of kidneys during surgery.
b) Endotoxic shock.
c) Obstructive jaundice.
d) Haemolytic transfusion reaction.
e) Long-standing renal disease.

16. Complications associated with acute pancreatitis include:
a) Toxic psychosis.
b) Jaundice.
c) Leucocytosis.
d) Cyanosis.
e) Hypercalcaemia.

17. Investigations useful in the diagnosis of obstructive jaundice are the following:
a) Endoscopic retrograde cholangiopancreatography.
b) Percutaneous transhepatic cholangiography.
c) Computed tomography.
d) Liver biopsy.
e) Ultrasonography.

18. Short stature with proportionate height is seen in the following:
a) Hypothyroidism.
b) Rickets.
c) Coeliac disease.
d) Malabsorption syndrome.
e) Achondroplasia.

19. Recognized features of subarachnoid haemorrhage include:
a) Epilepsy.
b) Paraplegia.
c) Hemiplegia.
d) Cranial nerve palsy.
e) Signs of meningism.

20. Firm swelling attached to the skin but not to the masseter muscle below can be due to:
   a) Lymph node.
   b) Sebaceous cyst.
   c) Pleomorphic adenoma.
   d) Adenolymphoma.
   e) Malignancy.

21. The following are infections which can be contracted by pets:
   a) Toxoplasmosis.
   b) Hydatid cyst.
   c) Toxocariasis.
   d) Tetanus.
   e) Tetany.

22. Recognized features of biliary cirrhosis include:
   a) Autoimmune mechanism.
   b) Obstructive jaundice.
   c) Acute renal failure.
   d) Pigmentation.
   e) Pruritus.

23. Hormonal treatment is useful in cancers of the following:
   a) Prostate.
   b) Lung.
   c) Colon.
   d) Breast.
   e) Ovary.

24. Lymphocytosis is associated with:
   a) Tuberculosis.
   b) Viral infection.
   c) Pyogenic infection.
   d) Meningococcaemia.
   e) Haemophilus influenza.

25. Recognized manifestations of increased alcohol intake include:
   a) Increased MCV.
   b) Thiamin deficiency.
   c) Cerebellar ataxia.
   d) Macrocytosis.
   e) Cardiomyopathy.

26. The following are sedative drugs:
   a) Heroin.
   b) Dimorphine.
   c) Tricyclic antidepressants.
   d) Diazepam.
   e) Propranalol.

27. Laceration with contamination can be treated with:
   a) Tetanus toxoid.
   b) Tetanus immunoglobulin.
   c) Debridement.
   d) Primary suture.
   e) Prophylactic antibiotic.

28. Recognized manifestations of diverticulosis include:
   a) Pneumaturia.
   b) Malignancy.
   c) Gastro-colic fistula.
   d) Colo-colic fistula.
   e) Stricture.

29. Radioactive iodine therapy:
   a) May result in hypothyroidism.
   b) May result in hypoparathyroidism.
   c) Can be given in pregnancy.
   d) Peptic ulceration is a recognized complication.
   e) Useful in the treatment of carcinoma of the thyroid.

30. Increased gastric secretion occurs with the following treatment:
a) Misoprostol.
b) Prednisolone.
c) Prostaglandin E.
d) Codeine phosphate.
e) Omeprazole.

31. The following features are associated with haemochromatosis:
a) Cardiac failure.
b) Sterility.
c) Impotence.
d) Chondrocalcinosis.
e) Hypoglycaemia.

32. Bladder carcinoma is associated with the following conditions:
a) Interstitial cystitis.
b) Diverticulitis of the bladder.
c) Smoking.
d) Aromatic amines.
e) Schistosomiasis haematobium infestation.

33. Intrauterine growth retardation is known to occur in:
a) Multiple pregnancy.
b) Pre-eclampsia.
c) Alcoholism.
d) Smoking.
e) Intrauterine infection.

34. A femoral pulse may not be felt in the following conditions:
a) Thromboangiitis obliterans.
b) Polyarteritis nodosa.
c) Leriche's syndrome.
d) Coarctation of the aorta.
e) Dissecting aneurysm.

35. **Which of the following are associated with intermittent claudication?:**
   a) Polycythaemia.
   b) Anaemia.
   c) Hyperthyroidism.
   d) Diabetes mellitus.
   e) Aneurysm of the aorta.

36. **Increased alpha-fetoprotein is known to occur in:**
   a) Hydatidiform mole.
   b) Down's syndrome.
   c) Pre-eclampsic toxaemia.
   d) Neural tube defects.
   e) Multiple pregnancy.

37. **Unstable lie may be associated with the following:**
   a) Multiple pregnancy.
   b) Oligohydramnios.
   c) Multiparity.
   d) Intrauterine tumour.
   e) Uterine anomaly.

38. **The following tests help in recognizing malnutrition:**
   a) Triceps fold measurement.
   b) Hypoalbuminaemia.
   c) Upper arm circumference measurement.
   d) Hypercalcaemia.
   e) Hyperkalaemia.

39. **Hallucinations are characteristic of the following conditions:**
   a) Obsessive compulsive disorder.
   b) Alcohol withdrawal.
   c) Schizophrenia.
   d) Sleep deprivation.
   e) Depression.

40. Pneumonia is a recognized complication of the following:
   a) Hepatitis B virus infection.
   b) Typhoid.
   c) Q fever.
   d) Rheumatic fever.
   e) AIDS.

41. In painful arc syndrome:
   a) There is a history of fracture of the humerus.
   b) The patient shows middle third abduction difficulty.
   c) Intravenous steroid is treatment of choice.
   d) The pathology is at the insertion of the tendon at greater tuberosity.
   e) NSAIDs are useful.

42. In a menstrual cycle of 35 days ovulation occurs at:
   a) Peak of oestrogen rise.
   b) Progesterone rise.
   c) Midcycle.
   d) 14 days before menstruation.
   e) 14 days after menstruation.

43. Epistaxis with reduced platelet count is known to occur in:
   a) Severe megaloblastic anaemia.
   b) Aplastic anaemia.
   c) Haemolytic anaemia.
   d) Acute myeloblastic anaemia.
   e) Hereditary telangiectasis.

44. In polymyalgia rheumatica:
   a) Pain in the fingers is an association.
   b) Headache may be associated.
   c) Mild to moderate splenomegaly is usually seen.
   d) ESR is typically very high.
   e) CK is markedly raised.

45. **Recognized causes of hyponatraemia include:**
    a) Cushing's syndrome.
    b) Chronic renal failure.
    c) Conn's syndrome.
    d) Head injury.
    e) Addison's disease.

46. **Recognized features of congenital adrenal hyperplasia include:**
    a) Adolescent hirsutism.
    b) Fetal virilization.
    c) Karyotype abnormality.
    d) 21-Hydroxylase deficiency.
    e) Accelerated growth.

47. **The following features are associated with myasthenia gravis:**
    a) Muscle wasting.
    b) Proximal muscle affection.
    c) Ocular muscle affection.
    d) Diplopia.
    e) Respiratory failure.

48. **Autoantibodies are found to be increased in the following:**
    a) Colloidal goitre.
    b) Chronic active hepatitis.
    c) Ulcerative colitis.
    d) Crohn's disease.
    e) Biliary cirrhosis.

49. **Gastric carcinoma is associated with the following conditions:**
    a) Smoking.
    b) Alcohol.
    c) *Helicobacter pylori.*
    d) Gastric polyp.
    e) Blood group A.

50. Characteristic features of Parkinsonism include:
   a) Reduced dopamine in substantia nigra.
   b) Clasp-knife rigidity.
   c) Changes in personality.
   d) Stereotactic speech.
   e) Hypokinesia.

51. Type 1 respiratory failure is known to occur in the following:
   a) Bronchiectasis.
   b) Fibrosing alveolitis.
   c) Acute left ventricular failure.
   d) Sarcoidosis.
   e) Pneumonia.

52. Left parasternal heave as a clinical sign is seen in:
   a) Mitral stenosis.
   b) Tricuspid stenosis.
   c) Tricuspid atresia.
   d) Ventricular septal defect.
   e) Aortic stenosis.

53. The following are recognized causes of eosinophilia:
   a) Parasitic infestation.
   b) Systemic lupus erythematosus.
   c) Motor neurone disease.
   d) Toxoplasmosis gondii.
   e) Rubella.

54. An increase in jugular venous pressure is associated with the following conditions:
   a) Cardiac tamponade.
   b) Pulmonary hypertension.
   c) Superior vena cava obstruction.
   d) Pericardial effusion.
   e) Constrictive pericarditis.

55. Causes of small muscle wasting include:
   a) Cervical rib.
   b) Multiple sclerosis.
   c) Cryoglobulinaemia.
   d) Motor neurone disease.
   e) Rheumatoid arthritis.

56. Recognized features associated with idiopathic thrombocytopenic purpura include:
   a) Increased bleeding time.
   b) Positive Hess test.
   c) Moderate splenomegaly.
   d) Self-limiting course.
   e) Splenectomy usually helpful.

57. The following features may be associated with acute rheumatoid arthritis:
   a) Posterior dislocation of tibia.
   b) Rapidly rising ESR.
   c) Synovial thickening.
   d) Ruptured patellar tendon.
   e) Sausage-shaped fingers.

58. Occipito-posterior position:
   a) Is often associated with android pelvis.
   b) Chin is the usual denominator.
   c) Delivery occurs with extension of the head.
   d) Occurs in 25% of pregnancies.
   e) In 73% spontaneous vaginal delivery occurs.

59. Anal carcinoma:
   a) Can be basaloid in histology.
   b) Characteristically involves inferior mesenteric lymph nodes.
   c) May be papillary columnar in nature.
   d) Can involve superficial inguinal lymph nodes.
   e) Usually squamous cell type.

60. Avascular necrosis of bone may be associated with the following conditions:
a) Compartmental syndrome.
b) Steroid therapy.
c) Trochanteric fracture.
d) Osteomalacia.
e) Rheumatoid arthritis.

Paper 1   Answers

1. a) True
b) True
c) True
d) False
e) False

2. a) True
b) True
c) True
d) True
e) True

3. a) True
b) False
c) True
d) False
e) True

4. a) True
b) True
c) True
d) False
e) False

5. a) True
b) True
c) True
d) False
e) True

6. a) True
b) True
c) False
d) True
e) True

7. a) True
b) False
c) True
d) True
e) False

8. a) False
b) True
c) False
d) True
e) True

9. a) False
b) True
c) False
d) True
e) True

10. a) True
b) True
c) True
d) True
e) False

11. a) True
b) False
c) True
d) False
e) True

12. a) True
b) True
c) True
d) True
e) True

13. a) False
b) True
c) False
d) True
e) False

14. a) False
b) True
c) False
d) True
e) True

15. a) False
b) True
c) True
d) True
e) True

16. a) False
   b) True
   c) False
   d) False
   e) True

17. a) False
   b) True
   c) True
   d) True
   e) True

18. a) False
   b) True
   c) False
   d) True
   e) False

19. a) True
   b) True
   c) True
   d) True
   e) False

20. a) True
   b) True
   c) True
   d) True
   e) True

21. a) True
   b) False
   c) True
   d) True
   e) False

22. a) False
   b) True
   c) True
   d) False
   e) False

23. a) True
   b) True
   c) True
   d) True
   e) False

24. a) True
   b) True
   c) True
   d) True
   e) False

25. a) True
   b) False
   c) True
   d) True
   e) False

26. a) True
   b) False
   c) False
   d) False
   e) True

27. a) False
   b) True
   c) True
   d) True
   e) True

28. a) True
   b) True
   c) False
   d) True
   e) True

29. a) True
   b) True
   c) True
   d) True
   e) True

30. a) True
   b) True
   c) True
   d) True
   e) False

31. a) False
   b) True
   c) True
   d) True
   e) True

32. a) True
   b) True
   c) True
   d) True
   e) False

33. a) False
   b) True
   c) True
   d) False
   e) True

34. a) False
b) True
c) True
d) True
e) True

35. a) True
b) True
c) False
d) True
e) True

36. a) False
b) True
c) True
d) False
e) True

37. a) True
b) False
c) True
d) True
e) True

38. a) True
b) True
c) True
d) False
e) True

39. a) False
b) True
c) False
d) False
e) True

40. a) True
b) False
c) False
d) False
e) False

41. a) True
b) False
c) True
d) False
e) True

42. a) True
b) True
c) True
d) False
e) False

43. a) True
b) True
c) False
d) True
e) False

44. a) False
b) True
c) True
d) True
e) True

45. a) True
b) False
c) True
d) False
e) True

46. a) True
b) True
c) True
d) True
e) True

47. a) True
b) True
c) True
d) True
e) False

48. a) True
b) True
c) False
d) True
e) True

49. a) True
b) True
c) True
d) False
e) True

50. a) True
b) True
c) True
d) False
e) True

51. a) True
b) True
c) False
d) False
e) True

52. a) True
b) True
c) True
d) False
e) True

53. a) False
b) True
c) True
d) False
e) False

54. a) True
b) True
c) False
d) True
e) True

55. a) False
b) True
c) True
d) True
e) True

56. a) True
b) True
c) True
d) False
e) False

57. a) True
b) True
c) False
d) True
e) False

58. a) False
b) False
c) True
d) False
e) False

59. a) False
b) True
c) False
d) True
e) False

60. a) False
b) True
c) False
d) False
e) False

Paper 2   Answers

1. a) True
   b) False
   c) False
   d) True
   e) True

2. a) True
   b) True
   c) False
   d) True
   e) True

3. a) False
   b) True
   c) True
   d) True
   e) True

4. a) True
   b) True
   c) False
   d) False
   e) True

5. a) True
   b) True
   c) False
   d) True
   e) True

6. a) True
   b) True
   c) True
   d) True
   e) False

7. a) True
   b) True
   c) True
   d) False
   e) False

8. a) True
   b) True
   c) True
   d) False
   e) False

9. a) True
   b) True
   c) False
   d) True
   e) True

10. a) True
   b) True
   c) True
   d) False
   e) True

11. a) True
   b) True
   c) False
   d) False
   e) False

12. a) False
   b) True
   c) False
   d) True
   e) False

13. a) True
   b) True
   c) True
   d) False
   e) True

14. a) False
   b) True
   c) True
   d) True
   e) True

15. a) True
   b) False
   c) True
   d) True
   e) True

16. a) True
   b) True
   c) False
   d) True
   e) True

17. a) False
   b) True
   c) True
   d) True
   e) False

18. a) False
   b) True
   c) False
   d) False
   e) True

19. a) True
   b) True
   c) False
   d) False
   e) True

20. a) False
   b) False
   c) True
   d) True
   e) True

21. a) False
   b) False
   c) False
   d) False
   e) True

22. a) True
   b) False
   c) False
   d) True
   e) True

23. a) True
   b) True
   c) False
   d) False
   e) True

24. a) True
   b) False
   c) True
   d) False
   e) True

25. a) False
   b) False
   c) False
   d) True
   e) True

26. a) True
   b) True
   c) True
   d) True
   e) False

27. a) True
   b) False
   c) False
   d) True
   e) True

28. a) True
   b) True
   c) True
   d) False
   e) True

29. a) True
   b) True
   c) True
   d) False
   e) False

30. a) True
   b) True
   c) True
   d) True
   e) False

31. a) True
   b) False
   c) False
   d) False
   e) False

32. a) True
   b) False
   c) True
   d) False
   e) False

33. a) False
   b) True
   c) True
   d) True
   e) True

34. a) True
    b) True
    c) True
    d) True
    e) True

35. a) False
    b) False
    c) False
    d) False
    e) True

36. a) False
    b) False
    c) True
    d) True
    e) True

37. a) True
    b) True
    c) True
    d) True
    e) True

38. a) False
    b) True
    c) False
    d) True
    e) False

39. a) False
    b) True
    c) True
    d) True
    e) True

40. a) True
    b) False
    c) True
    d) True
    e) True

41. a) True
    b) False
    c) True
    d) True
    e) True

42. a) False
    b) False
    c) False
    d) True
    e) True

43. a) True
    b) False
    c) False
    d) False
    e) True

44. a) True
    b) True
    c) False
    d) True
    e) True

45. a) True
    b) False
    c) True
    d) True
    e) True

46. a) False
    b) True
    c) False
    d) True
    e) False

47. a) True
    b) False
    c) False
    d) False
    e) False

48. a) True
    b) True
    c) True
    d) False
    e) True

49. a) False
    b) False
    c) True
    d) False
    e) True

50. a) True
    b) True
    c) True
    d) False
    e) True

51 a) False
   b) True
   c) False
   d) False
   e) True

52. a) False
b) True
c) True
d) False
e) False

53. a) True
b) False
c) True
d) True
e) True

54. a) True
b) True
c) False
d) True
e) False

55. a) False
b) False
c) False
d) False
e) True

56. a) True
b) True
c) False
d) False
e) True

57. a) True
b) True
c) True
d) False
e) False

58. a) True
b) True
c) True
d) True
e) True

59. a) False
b) False
c) True
d) True
e) True

60. a) False
b) True
c) True
d) True
e) True

Paper 3   Answers

1. a) False
b) False
c) False
d) True
e) True

2. a) False
b) True
c) False
d) True
e) False

3. a) False
b) True
c) True
d) True
e) True

4. a) False
b) True
c) True
d) True
e) False

5. a) False
b) False
c) True
d) True
e) False

6. a) True
b) True
c) False
d) True
e) True

7. a) True
b) False
c) False
d) False
e) False

8. a) True
b) True
c) False
d) False
e) False

9. a) True
b) True
c) False
d) True
e) True

10. a) True
b) True
c) False
d) True
e) True

11. a) False
b) True
c) True
d) True
e) True

12. a) True
b) False
c) False
d) True
e) False

13. a) False
b) True
c) False
d) True
e) True

14. a) False
b) True
c) False
d) True
e) True

15. a) True
b) True
c) False
d) True
e) True

16. a) True
b) True
c) True
d) True
e) False

17. a) True
b) False
c) True
d) False
e) False

18. a) True
b) True
c) True
d) True
e) True

19. a) False
b) True
c) True
d) True
e) True

20. a) False
b) False
c) True
d) False
e) False

21. a) True
b) True
c) True
d) False
e) False

22. a) True
b) True
c) True
d) True
e) True

23. a) True
b) True
c) True
d) False
e) True

24. a) False
b) True
c) False
d) False
e) False

25. a) True
b) True
c) False
d) False
e) True

26. a) True
b) True
c) True
d) True
e) True

27. a) True
b) False
c) False
d) True
e) False

28. a) True
b) True
c) False
d) False
e) False

29. a) False
b) True
c) True
d) False
e) True

30. a) True
b) True
c) True
d) True
e) True

31. a) True
b) False
c) True
d) False
e) False

32. a) True
b) True
c) True
d) False
e) False

33. a) False
b) False
c) False
d) True
e) False

34. a) False
b) True
c) False
d) False
e) False

35. a) True
b) True
c) False
d) False
e) True

36. a) False
b) False
c) True
d) True
e) False

37. a) True
b) False
c) False
d) False
e) False

38. a) True
b) False
c) False
d) False
e) False

39. a) False
b) False
c) True
d) True
e) False

40. a) True
b) False
c) True
d) False
e) True

41. a) False
b) True
c) True
d) True
e) True

42. a) True
b) True
c) False
d) False
e) True

43. a) True
b) True
c) True
d) True
e) True

44. a) False
b) True
c) True
d) True
e) True

45. a) False
b) False
c) False
d) False
e) True

46. a) True
b) False
c) True
d) False
e) True

47. a) False
b) False
c) True
d) False
e) False

48. a) False
b) True
c) True
d) True
e) True

49. a) True
b) False
c) False
d) True
e) False

50. a) True
b) True
c) False
d) True
e) False

51. a) True
b) True
c) False
d) False
e) False

52. a) True
b) False
c) True
d) True
e) True

53. a) True
b) False
c) True
d) False
e) True

54. a) True
b) True
c) False
d) True
e) False

55. a) False
b) True
c) False
d) True
e) True

56. a) False
b) False
c) True
d) True
e) False

57. a) True
b) False
c) True
d) False
e) True

58. a) True
b) False
c) True
d) True
e) False

59. a) False
b) True
c) True
d) False
e) True

60. a) True
b) False
c) False
d) False
e) True

Paper 4   Answers

1. a) True
   b) True
   c) False
   d) False
   e) True

2. a) True
   b) False
   c) False
   d) False
   e) True

3. a) False
   b) False
   c) True
   d) False
   e) False

4. a) False
   b) False
   c) True
   d) False
   e) False

5. a) False
   b) True
   c) True
   d) True
   e) True

6. a) True
   b) True
   c) False
   d) False
   e) False

7. a) True
   b) True
   c) False
   d) False
   e) True

8. a) True
   b) True
   c) False
   d) False
   e) False

9. a) True
   b) False
   c) False
   d) True
   e) True

10. a) True
   b) True
   c) False
   d) True
   e) True

11. a) True
   b) True
   c) True
   d) False
   e) True

12. a) True
   b) True
   c) True
   d) False
   e) False

13. a) True
   b) True
   c) False
   d) False
   e) False

14. a) False
   b) True
   c) True
   d) False
   e) True

15. a) True
   b) True
   c) False
   d) False
   e) True

16. a) False
b) True
c) False
d) True
e) False

17. a) False
b) True
c) True
d) False
e) True

18. a) False
b) True
c) True
d) True
e) True

19. a) False
b) False
c) False
d) True
e) False

20. a) True
b) False
c) True
d) True
e) True

21. a) True
b) False
c) True
d) True
e) True

22. a) False
b) True
c) True
d) False
e) False

23. a) True
b) True
c) False
d) False
e) True

24. a) False
b) True
c) True
d) False
e) True

25. a) True
b) True
c) True
d) False
e) False

26. a) True
b) True
c) True
d) True
e) False

27. a) True
b) True
c) False
d) True
e) True

28. a) False
b) False
c) False
d) True
e) True

29. a) True
b) False
c) False
d) False
e) False

30. a) True
b) False
c) True
d) True
e) False

31. a) False
b) True
c) True
d) True
e) True

32. a) True
b) True
c) False
d) False
e) True

33. a) False
b) True
c) False
d) False
e) False

34. a) False
b) False
c) True
d) False
e) False

35. a) True
b) True
c) True
d) False
e) True

36. a) False
b) True
c) False
d) False
e) True

37. a) True
b) False
c) True
d) False
e) True

38. a) True
b) True
c) True
d) False
e) True

39. a) False
b) True
c) True
d) True
e) True

40. a) False
b) True
c) False
d) True
e) False

41. a) True
b) True
c) False
d) False
e) False

42. a) True
b) True
c) True
d) True
e) True

43. a) False
b) True
c) False
d) True
e) True

44. a) True
b) False
c) True
d) True
e) True

45. a) True
b) True
c) False
d) True
e) False

46. a) True
b) True
c) False
d) False
e) False

47. a) True
b) True
c) True
d) True
e) True

48. a) False
b) False
c) True
d) False
e) True

49. a) False
b) True
c) True
d) True
e) True

50. a) False
b) True
c) False
d) False
e) False

51. a) True
b) False
c) False
d) True
e) True

52. a) True
b) True
c) True
d) False
e) True

53. a) True
b) False
c) True
d) True
e) True

54. a) True
b) True
c) True
d) True
e) False

55. a) True
b) False
c) False
d) False
e) True

56. a) False
b) True
c) True
d) False
e) True

57. a) True
b) True
c) True
d) False
e) True

58. a) False
b) False
c) True
d) True
e) False

59. a) False
b) False
c) True
d) False
e) True

60. a) True
b) True
c) True
d) False
e) True

Paper 5   Answers

1. a) True
b) True
c) False
d) True
e) True

2. a) False
b) False
c) False
d) False
e) False

3. a) True
b) False
c) False
d) True
e) True

4. a) True
b) False
c) True
d) True
e) False

5. a) False
b) True
c) True
d) False
e) True

6. a) True
b) True
c) False
d) False
e) True

7. a) True
b) False
c) False
d) True
e) True

8. a) True
b) True
c) True
d) True
e) True

9. a) True
b) True
c) False
d) True
e) True

10. a) True
b) True
c) False
d) False
e) True

11. a) True
b) True
c) True
d) False
e) True

12. a) True
b) True
c) True
d) True
e) True

13. a) True
b) True
c) False
d) False
e) False

14. a) True
b) True
c) True
d) False
e) True

15. a) True
b) False
c) False
d) False
e) True

16. a) True
b) False
c) True
d) True
e) True

17. a) True
b) False
c) False
d) True
e) True

18. a) False
b) False
c) True
d) True
e) True

19. a) True
b) True
c) False
d) True
e) True

20. a) False
b) False
c) True
d) True
e) False

21. a) False
b) True
c) True
d) False
e) True

22. a) False
b) True
c) False
d) True
e) True

23. a) True
b) False
c) True
d) True
e) True

24. a) False
b) False
c) True
d) True
e) True

25. a) True
b) False
c) True
d) False
e) True

26. a) True
b) False
c) True
d) False
e) False

27. a) True
b) True
c) False
d) False
e) False

28. a) False
b) True
c) True
d) False
e) True

29. a) True
b) True
c) False
d) False
e) True

30. a) False
b) True
c) False
d) False
e) True

31. a) True
b) False
c) True
d) False
e) False

32. a) False
b) True
c) False
d) True
e) True

33. a) True
b) True
c) True
d) True
e) True

34. a) True
b) True
c) True
d) False
e) False

35. a) True
b) True
c) False
d) True
e) True

36. a) False
b) False
c) False
d) True
e) True

37. a) True
b) True
c) True
d) False
e) True

38. a) True
b) True
c) False
d) True
e) True

39. a) True
b) True
c) True
d) True
e) False

40. a) True
b) True
c) True
d) True
e) False

41. a) True
b) True
c) True
d) False
e) True

42. a) True
b) True
c) False
d) False
e) True

43. a) True
b) True
c) False
d) False
e) False

44. a) True
b) True
c) True
d) False
e) False

45. a) False
b) True
c) True
d) False
e) False

46. a) True
b) True
c) False
d) False
e) False

47. a) False
b) True
c) False
d) False
e) True

48. a) False
b) True
c) True
d) False
e) True

49. a) True
b) True
c) True
d) False
e) True

50. a) False
b) False
c) False
d) False
e) True

51. a) True
b) False
c) False
d) False
e) False

52. a) False
b) True
c) True
d) False
e) False

53. a) True
b) False
c) True
d) True
e) True

54. a) True
b) True
c) False
d) True
e) True

55. a) True
b) True
c) False
d) True
e) False

56. a) True
b) True
c) True
d) False
e) False

57. a) True
b) False
c) True
d) True
e) False

58. a) True
b) True
c) True
d) False
e) True

59. a) True
b) True
c) False
d) False
e) False

60. a) True
b) True
c) False
d) False
e) False

Paper 6   Answers

1. a) True
b) True
c) True
d) False
e) True

2. a) True
b) True
c) True
d) True
e) True

3. a) True
b) False
c) False
d) True
e) True

4. a) True
b) True
c) False
d) True
e) True

5. a) True
b) True
c) True
d) False
e) False

6. a) True
b) False
c) True
d) True
e) True

7. a) False
b) True
c) False
d) False
e) True

8. a) False
b) Truc
c) True
d) False
e) True

9. a) False
b) True
c) False
d) True
e) True

10. a) True
b) True
c) False
d) True
e) False

11. a) False
b) False
c) False
d) True
e) True

12. a) True
b) True
c) True
d) False
e) True

13. a) True
b) False
c) True
d) False
e) False

14. a) True
b) True
c) False
d) True
e) True

15. a) True
b) True
c) True
d) False
e) True

16. a) True
b) False
c) True
d) True
e) True

17. a) True
b) True
c) False
d) True
e) False

18. a) False
b) False
c) True
d) True
e) False

19. a) False
b) True
c) False
d) False
e) False

20. a) True
b) True
c) False
d) False
e) True

21. a) True
b) True
c) True
d) True
e) True

22. a) False
b) True
c) True
d) True
e) True

23. a) True
b) True
c) False
d) True
e) False

24. a) True
b) True
c) False
d) True
e) True

25. a) True
b) True
c) True
d) False
e) True

26. a) True
b) True
c) False
d) True
e) True

27. a) True
b) True
c) True
d) True
e) True

28. a) True
b) True
c) True
d) False
e) True

29. a) False
b) True
c) False
d) True
e) True

30. a) True
b) False
c) False
d) True
e) True

31. a) True
b) True
c) False
d) True
e) True

32. a) True
b) True
c) True
d) True
e) True

33. a) False
b) False
c) False
d) False
e) False

34. a) True
b) False
c) True
d) False
e) False

35. a) True
b) True
c) True
d) True
e) True

36. a) True
b) True
c) False
d) True
e) True

37. a) True
b) False
c) False
d) True
e) True

38. a) False
b) True
c) False
d) False
e) False

39. a) False
b) False
c) True
d) True
e) True

40. a) True
b) True
c) True
d) False
e) False

41. a) False
b) False
c) True
d) True
e) True

42. a) True
b) False
c) False
d) True
e) False

43. a) False
b) True
c) False
d) False
e) False

44. a) True
b) True
c) True
d) True
e) True

45. a) False
b) False
c) False
d) True
e) False

46. a) True
b) True
c) True
d) True
e) False

47. a) False
b) False
c) True
d) True
e) True

48. a) True
b) True
c) True
d) True
e) True

49. a) True
b) True
c) True
d) True
e) True

50. a) True
b) True
c) False
d) True
e) True

51. a) True
b) True
c) True
d) True
e) False

52. a) False
b) False
c) True
d) True
e) False

53. a) True
b) True
c) False
d) False
e) True

54. a) True
b) True
c) False
d) False
e) False

55. a) False
b) False
c) False
d) True
e) False

56. a) True
b) True
c) False
d) True
e) False

57. a) True
b) False
c) True
d) True
e) True

58. a) False
b) True
c) True
d) True
e) True

59. a) False
b) False
c) False
d) False
e) True

60. a) True
b) True
c) True
d) True
e) False

Paper 7   Answers

1. a) True
   b) True
   c) True
   d) True
   e) True

2. a) True
   b) False
   c) False
   d) False
   e) True

3. a) False
   b) False
   c) True
   d) False
   e) False

4. a) True
   b) True
   c) True
   d) False
   e) True

5. a) True
   b) True
   c) True
   d) True
   e) True

6. a) False
   b) False
   c) True
   d) True
   e) True

7. a) True
   b) True
   c) True
   d) True
   e) True

8. a) True
   b) False
   c) True
   d) True
   e) False

9. a) False
   b) True
   c) False
   d) True
   e) True

10. a) True
   b) True
   c) True
   d) False
   e) True

11. a) True
   b) True
   c) True
   d) False
   e) True

12. a) True
   b) True
   c) False
   d) False
   e) False

13. a) False
   b) True
   c) True
   d) False
   e) False

14. a) True
   b) True
   c) True
   d) True
   e) True

15. a) False
   b) True
   c) True
   d) True
   e) True

16. a) True
b) True
c) False
d) True
e) False

17. a) False
b) True
c) True
d) False
e) False

18. a) False
b) True
c) False
d) True
e) True

19. a) False
b) True
c) True
d) True
e) True

20. a) True
b) True
c) False
d) True
e) True

21. a) True
b) False
c) True
d) False
e) True

22. a) True
b) True
c) True
d) True
e) False

23. a) True
b) True
c) True
d) False
e) False

24. a) True
b) True
c) True
d) False
e) False

25. a) True
b) True
c) True
d) True
e) True

26. a) True
b) True
c) True
d) True
e) True

27. a) True
b) False
c) True
d) False
e) True

28. a) True
b) True
c) True
d) True
e) True

29. a) True
b) False
c) True
d) False
e) True

30. a) True
b) True
c) False
d) True
e) True

31. a) True
b) False
c) True
d) True
e) False

32. a) False
b) False
c) False
d) False
e) True

33. a) True
b) False
c) False
d) False
e) False

34. a) False
b) False
c) False
d) False
e) True

35. a) False
b) False
c) True
d) True
e) True

36. a) False
b) True
c) False
d) False
e) True

37. a) True
b) True
c) True
d) True
e) True

38. a) False
b) True
c) True
d) True
e) True

39. a) False
b) True
c) True
d) True
e) False

40. a) True
b) False
c) True
d) True
e) False

41. a) False
b) False
c) True
d) False
e) True

42. a) False
b) True
c) True
d) False
e) False

43. a) False
b) True
c) False
d) True
e) False

44. a) True
b) True
c) True
d) False
e) True

45. a) True
b) False
c) True
d) True
e) False

46. a) True
b) False
c) True
d) True
e) False

47. a) True
b) True
c) False
d) False
e) False

48. a) True
b) False
c) True
d) False
e) True

49. a) False
b) False
c) True
d) False
e) True

50. a) True
b) True
c) True
d) False
e) False

51. a) False
b) True
c) False
d) False
e) False

52. a) False
b) True
c) False
d) False
e) True

53. a) False
b) True
c) True
d) True
e) False

54. a) False
b) True
c) False
d) True
e) True

55. a) False
b) False
c) True
d) True
e) True

56. a) False
b) False
c) True
d) True
e) True

57. a) True
b) True
c) True
d) False
e) False

58. a) True
b) False
c) True
d) True
e) False

59. a) False
b) True
c) True
d) True
e) True

60. a) True
b) True
c) True
d) True
e) True

Paper 8   Answers

1. a) True
    b) True
    c) True
    d) True
    e) False

2. a) True
    b) True
    c) True
    d) True
    e) True

3. a) True
    b) True
    c) False
    d) True
    e) True

4. a) False
    b) True
    c) True
    d) True
    e) True

5. a) False
    b) True
    c) True
    d) True
    e) True

6. a) True
    b) True
    c) True
    d) True
    e) True

7. a) True
    b) True
    c) True
    d) False
    e) True

8. a) True
    b) True
    c) True
    d) True
    e) False

9. a) False
    b) False
    c) True
    d) False
    e) True

10. a) False
    b) False
    c) True
    d) False
    e) True

11. a) True
    b) True
    c) False
    d) False
    e) True

12. a) True
    b) True
    c) False
    d) False
    e) False

13. a) False
    b) True
    c) False
    d) True
    e) False

14. a) True
    b) True
    c) True
    d) True
    e) True

15. a) False
    b) True
    c) False
    d) True
    e) True

16. a) True
b) False
c) True
d) True
e) True

17. a) True
b) False
c) False
d) False
e) False

18. a) True
b) True
c) True
d) True
e) True

19. a) True
b) True
c) True
d) True
e) False

20. a) True
b) True
c) True
d) True
e) True

21. a) False
b) True
c) False
d) False
e) False

22. a) True
b) True
c) True
d) False
e) True

23. a) False
b) True
c) True
d) True
e) True

24. a) True
b) True
c) False
d) True
e) True

25. a) True
b) True
c) True
d) True
e) True

26. a) False
b) True
c) True
d) True
e) True

27. a) True
b) True
c) True
d) True
e) True

28. a) True
b) True
c) True
d) False
e) True

29. a) False
b) True
c) False
d) False
e) False

30. a) False
b) True
c) True
d) True
e) False

31. a) True
b) True
c) True
d) False
e) True

32. a) True
b) True
c) True
d) True
e) True

33. a) False
b) True
c) False
d) True
e) False

34. a) True
    b) False
    c) True
    d) False
    e) True

35. a) True
    b) True
    c) True
    d) True
    e) False

36. a) True
    b) True
    c) True
    d) False
    e) False

37. a) True
    b) False
    c) True
    d) False
    e) False

38. a) False
    b) False
    c) True
    d) False
    e) False

39. a) True
    b) True
    c) False
    d) True
    e) False

40. a) True
    b) True
    c) True
    d) False
    e) True

41. a) True
    b) True
    c) True
    d) True
    e) True

42. a) True
    b) True
    c) True
    d) True
    e) True

43. a) True
    b) True
    c) True
    d) False
    e) False

44. a) False
    b) True
    c) True
    d) False
    e) False

45. a) True
    b) True
    c) True
    d) True
    e) True

46. a) True
    b) False
    c) False
    d) False
    e) True

47. a) True
    b) True
    c) False
    d) True
    e) False

48. a) True
    b) False
    c) True
    d) True
    e) True

49. a) True
    b) True
    c) True
    d) True
    e) True

50. a) True
    b) True
    c) True
    d) True
    e) False

51. a) True
    b) True
    c) True
    d) True
    e) True

52. a) True
b) True
c) True
d) True
e) True

53. a) True
b) False
c) True
d) True
e) True

54. a) False
b) True
c) False
d) True
e) False

55. a) True
b) True
c) True
d) True
e) True

56. a) True
b) True
c) False
d) False
e) False

57. a) False
b) True
c) True
d) False
e) True

58. a) True
b) False
c) False
d) True
e) False

59. a) False
b) True
c) True
d) True
e) True

60. a) False
b) True
c) False
d) False
e) True

Paper 9   Answers

1. a) True
   b) False
   c) False
   d) True
   e) False

2. a) True
   b) False
   c) True
   d) False
   e) False

3. a) True
   b) False
   c) True
   d) False
   e) False

4. a) True
   b) True
   c) True
   d) True
   e) False

5. a) True
   b) False
   c) False
   d) True
   e) True

6. a) True
   b) True
   c) False
   d) False
   e) True

7. a) True
   b) True
   c) True
   d) False
   e) True

8. a) True
   b) False
   c) True
   d) True
   e) True

9. a) True
   b) False
   c) True
   d) True
   e) True

10. a) True
   b) True
   c) True
   d) True
   e) True

11. a) True
   b) False
   c) True
   d) False
   e) True

12. a) False
   b) False
   c) False
   d) True
   e) True

13. a) False
   b) True
   c) True
   d) False
   e) True

14. a) False
   b) True
   c) False
   d) True
   e) True

15. a) True
   b) False
   c) True
   d) False
   e) True

16. a) True
   b) False
   c) False
   d) True
   e) True

17. a) False
   b) True
   c) True
   d) True
   e) True

18. a) True
   b) True
   c) True
   d) False
   e) False

19. a) True
   b) True
   c) True
   d) True
   e) True

20. a) True
   b) True
   c) True
   d) True
   e) True

21. a) False
   b) True
   c) False
   d) True
   e) False

22. a) True
   b) True
   c) True
   d) False
   e) True

23. a) False
   b) True
   c) False
   d) False
   e) True

24. a) True
   b) True
   c) False
   d) False
   e) False

25. a) True
   b) True
   c) False
   d) True
   e) True

26. a) False
   b) True
   c) True
   d) True
   e) False

27. a) False
   b) True
   c) True
   d) True
   e) False

28. a) True
   b) False
   c) True
   d) False
   e) False

29. a) True
   b) False
   c) False
   d) False
   e) False

30. a) False
   b) True
   c) True
   d) True
   e) True

31. a) False
   b) True
   c) False
   d) False
   e) True

32. a) False
   b) False
   c) False
   d) True
   e) True

33. a) False
   b) True
   c) True
   d) True
   e) True

34. a) True
b) False
c) True
d) True
e) True

35. a) True
b) False
c) False
d) False
e) False

36. a) False
b) True
c) False
d) False
e) False

37. a) False
b) True
c) False
d) False
e) False

38. a) False
b) False
c) True
d) False
e) True

39. a) False
b) True
c) True
d) True
e) True

40. a) True
b) False
c) True
d) False
e) True

41. a) True
b) False
c) True
d) True
e) False

42. a) False
b) False
c) False
d) True
e) True

43. a) True
b) False
c) True
d) False
e) True

44. a) True
b) False
c) False
d) True
e) True

45. a) True
b) False
c) True
d) True
e) False

46. a) False
b) False
c) True
d) True
e) False

47. a) True
b) True
c) False
d) False
e) True

48. a) True
b) True
c) True
d) False
e) False

49. a) False
b) False
c) True
d) True
e) False

50. a) True
b) False
c) False
d) False
e) False

51. a) True
b) True
c) True
d) False
e) False

52. a) False
b) True
c) False
d) False
e) True

53. a) True
b) True
c) False
d) False
e) True

54. a) True
b) True
c) True
d) True
e) True

55. a) True
b) True
c) True
d) True
e) True

56. a) False
b) True
c) False
d) True
e) False

57. a) True
b) True
c) True
d) False
e) False

58. a) True
b) False
c) True
d) True
e) False

59. a) True
b) False
c) False
d) False
e) False

60. a) False
b) True
c) False
d) True
e) True

Paper 10   Answers

1. a) False
   b) True
   c) True
   d) False
   e) True

2. a) False
   b) True
   c) False
   d) True
   e) False

3. a) True
   b) True
   c) False
   d) False
   e) False

4. a) True
   b) True
   c) True
   d) False
   e) True

5. a) True
   b) True
   c) True
   d) True
   e) False

6. a) True
   b) False
   c) False
   d) True
   e) False

7. a) True
   b) True
   c) True
   d) True
   e) True

8. a) True
   b) True
   c) True
   d) False
   e) False

9. a) True
   b) False
   c) True
   d) True
   e) False

10. a) False
   b) True
   c) True
   d) False
   e) True

11. a) False
   b) True
   c) True
   d) False
   e) True

12. a) False
   b) True
   c) True
   d) False
   e) True

13. a) True
   b) True
   c) True
   d) True
   e) True

14. a) True
   b) True
   c) True
   d) True
   e) True

15. a) True
   b) True
   c) False
   d) True
   e) True

16. a) True
b) True
c) True
d) False
e) True

17. a) True
b) False
c) True
d) False
e) False

18. a) True
b) False
c) True
d) True
e) True

19. a) True
b) True
c) True
d) False
e) True

20. a) True
b) False
c) True
d) True
e) False

21. a) True
b) False
c) True
d) True
e) True

22. a) False
b) True
c) True
d) True
e) True

23. a) True
b) True
c) True
d) True
e) True

24. a) True
b) True
c) True
d) False
e) True

25. a) True
b) True
c) True
d) False
e) True

26. a) False
b) True
c) True
d) False
e) True

27. a) False
b) True
c) True
d) True
e) True

28. a) True
b) True
c) True
d) True
e) False

29. a) True
b) True
c) True
d) True
e) False

30. a) True
b) True
c) True
d) False
e) True

31. a) False
b) False
c) True
d) True
e) True

32. a) True
b) True
c) False
d) False
e) False

33. a) True
b) False
c) True
d) True
e) False

34. a) True
b) False
c) False
d) True
e) True

35. a) True
b) False
c) True
d) True
e) True

36. a) True
b) True
c) True
d) True
e) True

37. a) False
b) False
c) True
d) False
e) False

38. a) False
b) False
c) True
d) False
e) False

39. a) False
b) True
c) True
d) True
e) True

40. a) True
b) False
c) True
d) True
e) True

41. a) True
b) False
c) True
d) False
e) False

42. a) True
b) False
c) True
d) True
e) True

43. a) True
b) True
c) False
d) True
e) True

44. a) True
b) False
c) True
d) True
e) True

45. a) True
b) True
c) True
d) False
e) True

46. a) True
b) True
c) True
d) False
e) True

47. a) True
b) True
c) False
d) False
e) True

48. a) False
b) True
c) True
d) True
e) False

49. a) True
b) False
c) True
d) True
e) False

50. a) False
b) False
c) True
d) True
e) True

51. a) True
b) False
c) False
d) True
e) True

52. a) False
b) True
c) False
d) True
e) True

53. a) True
b) True
c) True
d) True
e) True

54. a) False
b) False
c) True
d) True
e) False

55. a) True
b) True
c) True
d) True
e) False

56. a) False
b) True
c) True
d) False
e) False

57. a) True
b) False
c) False
d) True
e) True

58. a) False
b) True
c) False
d) False
e) True

59. a) True
b) True
c) False
d) False
e) True

60. a) False
b) True
c) False
d) True
e) False

Paper 11   Answers

1. a) False
   b) False
   c) True
   d) True
   e) True

2. a) False
   b) True
   c) True
   d) True
   e) False

3. a) True
   b) False
   c) True
   d) True
   e) True

4. a) True
   b) False
   c) True
   d) False
   e) True

5. a) True
   b) True
   c) True
   d) True
   e) True

6. a) False
   b) True
   c) True
   d) False
   e) False

7. a) True
   b) True
   c) False
   d) False
   e) True

8. a) False
   b) True
   c) True
   d) True
   e) True

9. a) True
   b) False
   c) True
   d) True
   e) True

10. a) True
    b) True
    c) True
    d) False
    e) False

11. a) True
    b) False
    c) True
    d) True
    e) True

12. a) True
    b) True
    c) True
    d) True
    e) False

13. a) True
    b) False
    c) False
    d) False
    e) True

14. a) True
    b) True
    c) False
    d) True
    e) False

15. a) True
    b) True
    c) False
    d) True
    e) False

16. a) False
b) True
c) False
d) False
e) True

17. a) True
b) True
c) False
d) True
e) False

18. a) True
b) True
c) True
d) False
e) True

19. a) True
b) True
c) False
d) False
e) False

20. a) False
b) True
c) True
d) True
e) True

21. a) True
b) True
c) False
d) False
e) False

22. a) True
b) False
c) True
d) True
e) True

23. a) True
b) True
c) True
d) False
e) True

24. a) False
b) False
c) True
d) True
e) True

25. a) True
b) True
c) False
d) True
e) True

26. a) True
b) True
c) True
d) False
e) True

27. a) True
b) False
c) True
d) True
e) True

28. a) True
b) True
c) False
d) True
e) True

29. a) False
b) True
c) False
d) True
e) True

30. a) True
b) False
c) True
d) True
e) False

31. a) True
b) True
c) True
d) False
e) True

32. a) True
b) True
c) False
d) False
e) True

33. a) False
b) False
c) True
d) False
e) True

34. a) True
b) False
c) True
d) True
e) False

35. a) True
b) False
c) True
d) True
e) False

36. a) True
b) True
c) True
d) True
e) True

37. a) True
b) True
c) True
d) False
e) False

38. a) True
b) False
c) False
d) True
e) False

39. a) False
b) False
c) True
d) True
e) True

40. a) True
b) True
c) True
d) True
e) False

41. a) False
b) False
c) True
d) False
e) True

42. a) False
b) True
c) False
d) True
e) True

43. a) True
b) False
c) True
d) True
e) True

44. a) True
b) False
c) True
d) True
e) False

45. a) False
b) True
c) False
d) False
e) False

46. a) False
b) True
c) False
d) True
e) True

47. a) False
b) False
c) True
d) True
e) True

48. a) False
b) True
c) True
d) False
e) True

49. a) False
b) False
c) True
d) True
e) False

50. a) False
b) True
c) True
d) True
e) True

51. a) False
b) True
c) False
d) True
e) False

52. a) True
   b) False
   c) True
   d) True
   e) True

53. a) False
   b) False
   c) True
   d) True
   e) True

54. a) False
   b) True
   c) False
   d) False
   e) True

55. a) False
   b) False
   c) True
   d) False
   e) False

56. a) True
   b) False
   c) True
   d) False
   e) True

57. a) True
   b) True
   c) False
   d) False
   e) True

58. a) True
   b) True
   c) False
   d) True
   e) False

59. a) False
   b) False
   c) True
   d) True
   e) True

60. a) True
   b) False
   c) True
   d) False
   e) True

Paper 12 Answers

1. a) False
   b) True
   c) False
   d) False
   e) False

2. a) True
   b) False
   c) True
   d) False
   e) True

3. a) False
   b) True
   c) False
   d) False
   e) False

4. a) False
   b) True
   c) True
   d) False
   e) False

5. a) True
   b) False
   c) True
   d) False
   e) False

6. a) True
   b) False
   c) False
   d) True
   e) True

7. a) False
   b) True
   c) True
   d) True
   e) True

8. a) True
   b) False
   c) True
   d) False
   e) False

9. a) True
   b) True
   c) True
   d) False
   e) False

10. a) True
   b) True
   c) False
   d) True
   e) False

11. a) True
   b) True
   c) False
   d) False
   e) True

12. a) False
   b) True
   c) True
   d) False
   e) True

13. a) True
   b) True
   c) False
   d) True
   e) True

14. a) True
   b) False
   c) True
   d) True
   e) False

15. a) False
   b) False
   c) True
   d) True
   e) False

16. a) True
b) True
c) False
d) False
e) True

17. a) False
b) True
c) True
d) False
e) True

18. a) True
b) True
c) False
d) True
e) True

19. a) False
b) False
c) False
d) False
e) False

20. a) True
b) True
c) True
d) False
e) False

21. a) False
b) False
c) False
d) True
e) False

22. a) False
b) False
c) False
d) False
e) False

23. a) False
b) True
c) False
d) False
e) True

24. a) True
b) True
c) False
d) False
e) True

25. a) True
b) False
c) True
d) True
e) True

26. a) False
b) True
c) False
d) True
e) False

27. a) True
b) True
c) True
d) True
e) True

28. a) True
b) True
c) True
d) True
e) True

29. a) True
b) False
c) True
d) False
e) False

30. a) False
b) False
c) False
d) True
e) False

31. a) False
b) False
c) True
d) True
e) True

32. a) False
b) True
c) False
d) True
e) True

33. a) False
b) True
c) True
d) True
e) True

34. a) True
b) False
c) True
d) True
e) False

35. a) True
b) True
c) False
d) True
e) False

36. a) True
b) True
c) False
d) False
e) False

37. a) True
b) True
c) False
d) False
e) False

38. a) True
b) True
c) False
d) True
e) False

39. a) True
b) False
c) False
d) False
e) False

40. a) True
b) True
c) True
d) False
e) False

41. a) False
b) True
c) True
d) False
e) True

42. a) True
b) True
c) False
d) True
e) True

43. a) True
b) True
c) True
d) False
e) False

44. a) True
b) False
c) False
d) True
e) True

45. a) False
b) True
c) False
d) True
e) False

46. a) False
b) True
c) False
d) True
e) False

47. a) False
b) True
c) True
d) True
e) False

48. a) False
b) True
c) False
d) False
e) False

49. a) True
b) True
c) True
d) True
e) True

50. a) True
b) True
c) False
d) True
e) False

51. a) True
b) False
c) True
d) False
e) True

52. a) True
b) True
c) False
d) False
e) False

53. a) False
b) True
c) True
d) False
e) True

54. a) True
b) False
c) True
d) False
e) True

55. a) True
b) False
c) False
d) True
e) True

56. a) True
b) False
c) True
d) False
e) False

57. a) False
b) False
c) False
d) True
e) True

58. a) True
b) True
c) False
d) True
e) False

59. a) True
b) True
c) False
d) False
e) False

60. a) True
b) True
c) True
d) False
e) True

Paper 13   Answers

1. a) True
   b) False
   c) True
   d) True
   e) False

2. a) False
   b) True
   c) False
   d) True
   e) False

3. a) True
   b) True
   c) True
   d) False
   e) True

4. a) True
   b) True
   c) False
   d) False
   e) True

5. a) True
   b) False
   c) True
   d) True
   e) False

6. a) True
   b) False
   c) False
   d) True
   e) False

7. a) True
   b) False
   c) False
   d) True
   e) True

8. a) True
   b) True
   c) True
   d) False
   e) True

9. a) True
   b) True
   c) True
   d) False
   e) False

10. a) True
   b) True
   c) False
   d) False
   e) True

11. a) True
   b) False
   c) True
   d) True
   e) False

12. a) True
   b) True
   c) True
   d) False
   e) True

13. a) True
   b) False
   c) False
   d) False
   e) False

14. a) False
   b) True
   c) False
   d) True
   e) False

15. a) False
   b) False
   c) True
   d) False
   e) True

16. a) True
    b) False
    c) True
    d) True
    e) False

17. a) True
    b) False
    c) True
    d) False
    e) True

18. a) True
    b) True
    c) False
    d) False
    e) True

19. a) True
    b) True
    c) False
    d) True
    e) False

20. a) True
    b) False
    c) True
    d) False
    e) False

21. a) True
    b) True
    c) True
    d) True
    e) False

22. a) True
    b) True
    c) False
    d) True
    e) True

23. a) True
    b) False
    c) True
    d) True
    e) False

24. a) False
    b) True
    c) True
    d) True
    e) True

25. a) True
    b) True
    c) False
    d) True
    e) False

26. a) False
    b) False
    c) False
    d) True
    e) True

27. a) True
    b) True
    c) True
    d) True
    e) True

28. a) True
    b) True
    c) False
    d) True
    e) False

29. a) True
    b) False
    c) True
    d) True
    e) False

30. a) False
    b) True
    c) True
    d) True
    e) True

31. a) True
    b) True
    c) False
    d) False
    e) True

32. a) False
    b) False
    c) False
    d) False
    e) False

33. a) False
    b) True
    c) False
    d) False
    e) True

34. a) False
b) True
c) False
d) True
e) False

35. a) True
b) False
c) False
d) False
e) True

36. a) False
b) True
c) True
d) True
e) False

37. a) False
b) True
c) True
d) False
e) True

38. a) False
b) True
c) True
d) True
e) True

39. a) False
b) False
c) True
d) True
e) True

40. a) True
b) False
c) True
d) False
e) False

41. a) False
b) True
c) False
d) False
e) False

42. a) True
b) True
c) False
d) True
e) True

43. a) True
b) True
c) True
d) True
e) True

44. a) True
b) True
c) True
d) True
e) False

45. a) True
b) True
c) True
d) False
e) False

46. a) True
b) True
c) True
d) True
e) True

47. a) True
b) False
c) True
d) True
e) False

48. a) False
b) True
c) False
d) False
e) True

49. a) False
b) True
c) True
d) Truc
e) True

50. a) False
b) True
c) True
d) True
e) True

51. a) True
b) True
c) True
d) False
e) True

52. a) True
b) False
c) False
d) True
e) False

53. a) True
b) False
c) True
d) False
e) False

54. a) True
b) True
c) True
d) False
e) True

55. a) True
b) False
c) False
d) True
e) True

56. a) True
b) True
c) True
d) False
e) True

57. a) False
b) False
c) True
d) True
e) True

58. a) False
b) False
c) True
d) True
e) False

59. a) True
b) True
c) False
d) True
e) True

60. a) True
b) False
c) False
d) True
e) False

Paper 14   Answers

1. a) True
b) True
c) False
d) False
e) True

2. a) False
b) True
c) False
d) False
e) False

3. a) True
b) False
c) True
d) True
e) True

4. a) True
b) False
c) False
d) True
e) True

5. a) False
b) True
c) True
d) False
e) True

6. a) False
b) True
c) True
d) False
e) True

7. a) True
b) True
c) False
d) True
e) False

8. a) True
b) True
c) False
d) False
e) True

9. a) False
b) True
c) False
d) True
e) True

10. a) True
b) True
c) False
d) True
e) True

11. a) False
b) False
c) True
d) True
e) False

12. a) True
b) True
c) False
d) True
e) True

13. a) False
b) True
c) False
d) True
e) False

14. a) True
b) True
c) False
d) False
e) True

15. a) False
b) True
c) False
d) True
e) False

16. a) True
b) True
c) True
d) False
e) True

17. a) True
b) True
c) True
d) True
e) False

18. a) True
b) True
c) False
d) False
e) False

19. a) True
b) True
c) True
d) True
e) False

20. a) False
b) True
c) True
d) True
e) True

21. a) False
b) False
c) True
d) False
e) False

22. a) False
b) True
c) False
d) False
e) True

23. a) True
b) True
c) True
d) True
e) True

24. a) False
b) True
c) True
d) True
e) False

25. a) False
b) True
c) False
d) False
e) True

26. a) False
b) True
c) False
d) True
e) True

27. a) False
b) False
c) False
d) False
e) True

28. a) True
b) True
c) False
d) True
e) False

29. a) True
b) True
c) True
d) False
e) True

30. a) True
b) True
c) True
d) False
e) False

31. a) True
b) False
c) True
d) True
e) True

32. a) False
b) True
c) False
d) True
e) False

33. a) True
b) True
c) False
d) False
e) False

34. a) True
b) True
c) True
d) True
e) False

35. a) True
b) False
c) False
d) False
e) True

36. a) True
b) False
c) False
d) True
e) False

37. a) True
b) True
c) True
d) True
e) True

38. a) True
b) True
c) True
d) False
e) True

39. a) True
b) True
c) True
d) True
e) False

40. a) True
b) True
c) True
d) True
e) True

41. a) False
b) True
c) False
d) False
e) False

42. a) False
b) True
c) True
d) False
e) False

43. a) True
b) True
c) False
d) True
e) True

44. a) True
b) False
c) True
d) False
e) False

45. a) False
b) False
c) False
d) True
e) False

46. a) False
b) False
c) True
d) True
e) False

47. a) False
b) True
c) True
d) False
e) True

48. a) True
b) False
c) True
d) False
e) False

49. a) True
b) False
c) True
d) True
e) False

50. a) False
b) True
c) True
d) False
e) False

51. a) False
b) True
c) True
d) True
e) True

52. a) False
b) False
c) True
d) False
e) True

53. a) True
b) True
c) True
d) False
e) False

54. a) True
b) True
c) False
d) False
e) False

55. a) True
b) False
c) False
d) False
e) True

56. a) True
b) True
c) True
d) False
e) True

57. a) False
b) True
c) True
d) False
e) True

58. a) True
b) False
c) False
d) False
e) False

59. a) True
b) True
c) False
d) False
e) False

60. a) False
b) False
c) True
d) False
e) True

Paper 15   Answers

1. a) False
   b) True
   c) True
   d) True
   e) False

2. a) False
   b) True
   c) True
   d) True
   e) True

3. a) True
   b) True
   c) False
   d) True
   e) False

4. a) True
   b) False
   c) True
   d) False
   e) True

5. a) True
   b) True
   c) True
   d) True
   e) True

6. a) False
   b) True
   c) True
   d) True
   e) True

7. a) True
   b) False
   c) True
   d) False
   e) True

8. a) False
   b) True
   c) True
   d) True
   e) True

9. a) False
   b) True
   c) False
   d) True
   e) True

10. a) True
   b) True
   c) True
   d) True
   e) True

11. a) True
   b) False
   c) True
   d) False
   e) False

12. a) False
   b) True
   c) True
   d) False
   e) True

13. a) False
   b) True
   c) True
   d) True
   e) False

14. a) True
   b) False
   c) True
   d) True
   e) True

15. a) True
   b) True
   c) False
   d) True
   e) True

16. a) True
b) True
c) True
d) False
e) False

17. a) True
b) True
c) True
d) True
e) True

18. a) True
b) True
c) True
d) True
e) False

19. a) True
b) False
c) True
d) True
e) True

20. a) True
b) True
c) True
d) False
e) False

21. a) True
b) True
c) True
d) False
e) False

22. a) True
b) True
c) False
d) True
e) True

23. a) True
b) False
c) False
d) True
e) False

24. a) True
b) True
c) False
d) False
e) False

25. a) True
b) True
c) True
d) True
e) True

26. a) True
b) True
c) True
d) True
e) False

27. a) True
b) True
c) True
d) False
e) True

28. a) True
b) False
c) True
d) True
e) True

29. a) True
b) False
c) False
d) False
e) True

30. a) False
b) True
c) True
d) True
e) False

31. a) True
b) True
c) True
d) True
e) False

32. a) False
b) True
c) True
d) True
e) True

33. a) True
b) True
c) False
d) True
e) True

34. a) False
b) False
c) True
d) True
e) True

35. a) False
b) False
c) False
d) True
e) False

36. a) False
b) False
c) False
d) True
e) True

37. a) False
b) False
c) True
d) True
e) True

38. a) True
b) True
c) True
d) False
e) False

39. a) False
b) True
c) True
d) False
e) False

40. a) False
b) True
c) True
d) False
e) True

41. a) False
b) True
c) False
d) True
e) True

42. a) True
b) False
c) True
d) True
e) False

43. a) True
b) True
c) False
d) True
e) False

44. a) False
b) True
c) False
d) True
e) False

45. a) False
b) True
c) False
d) True
e) True

46. a) True
b) True
c) False
d) True
e) True

47. a) True
b) True
c) True
d) True
e) True

48. a) False
b) True
c) False
d) False
e) True

49. a) True
b) False
c) True
d) True
e) True

50. a) True
b) False
c) False
d) False
e) True

51. a) False
b) True
c) True
d) True
e) True

52. a) True
b) False
c) False
d) True
e) False

53. a) True
b) False
c) False
d) True
e) True

54. a) True
b) True
c) True
d) False
e) True

55. a) False
b) True
c) False
d) True
e) True

56. a) True
b) False
c) False
d) True
e) True

57. a) False
b) True
c) True
d) True
e) True

58. a) True
b) False
c) False
d) False
e) True

59. a) True
b) False
c) False
d) True
e) True

60. a) False
b) True
c) True
d) False
e) True

Index

N.B. Page references to questions and answers are prefixed by 'q' and 'a' respectively.

261